Knowledge for Nursing Practice

DATE DUE

Remembering
Andrew

Knowledge for Nursing Practice

Kate Robinson
PhD, BA, RGN, RHV
Dean of Health Care and Social Studies,
Luton College of Higher Education,
Luton, UK

and

Barbara Vaughan
MSc, RGN, DipN, DANS, RNT
Programme Director for Nursing Developments,
King's Fund Centre, London, UK

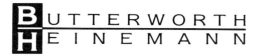

Butterworth-Heinemann Ltd
Linacre House, Jordan Hill, Oxford OX2 8DP

 PART OF REED INTERNATIONAL BOOKS

OXFORD   LONDON   BOSTON
MUNICH   NEW DELHI   SINGAPORE   SYDNEY
TOKYO   TORONTO   WELLINGTON

First published 1992

British Library Cataloguing in Publication Data
Robinson, Kate
    Knowledge for nursing practice.
    I. Title   II. Vaughan, Barbara
    610.73

ISBN 0 7506 0414 X

Printed and bound in Great Britain by Biddles Ltd, Guildford and Kings Lynn

Contents

Contributors

Philip Burnard PhD, MSc, RGN, RMN, DipN, CertEd

Philip Burnard is Director of Postgraduate Nursing Studies at the University of Wales College of Medicine and an honorary lecturer in nursing at the Hogeschool Middem Nederland, Utrecht, Netherlands. His research interests include experiential learning, counselling and interpersonal skills training in nursing.

Elisabeth Clark BA, PhD

Elisabeth Clark is currently a principal lecturer in the newly formed School of Health Care Studies, Middlesex Polytechnic. In this post she has responsibility for open learning and for teaching research awareness, research methods and statistics. Previously she was Director of the Distance Learning Centre (DLC), South Bank Polytechnic.

David Cook BA(Arizona), MA(Ed.), PhD(Ed.), MA(Oxon)

David Cook is currently Director of the Whitefield Institute and Fellow of Green College Oxford, teaches theology and ethics in the Theology Faculty and has responsibility for the teaching of medical ethics in the Medical Faculty. During his time in the States he was consultant to the United States government on the Black Power Movement.

Basiro Davey BSc, PhD

Basiro Davey is Lecturer in Health Studies at The Open University's Department of Biology in Milton Keynes. She was formerly a research immunologist working on the interaction of the immune system with cancer cells. She is currently chairing a multidisciplinary course team working on updating one of the Open University's most popular courses, *Health and Disease*, which attracts several hundred nurses each year among its students.

Mary FitzGerald MN, RGN, DipN (Lond.), CertEd

Mary Fitzgerald is currently working as a lecturer practitioner on the medical unit at the John Radcliffe Hospital in Oxford. She has a long clinical experience and held sister posts in general surgery, medicine and intensive care. She has also worked as a nurse tutor. In her present post she has responsibility for the nursing on an acute medical unit and for teaching the theory and practice of nursing for undergraduate students from a clinical basis.

Peter George BSc(Econ), MSc(Econ)

Peter George is Dean of Life Sciences at Oxford Polytechnic, has been a teacher of sociology and social policy in the sociology field and in a wide range of professional courses for more than twenty years. His main academic interests are in comparative social policy, welfare ideology and citizenship, but he also has a long-standing interest in the theory and practice of education for the health and social care professions. He was Co-Director of the team which designed the Polytechnic's Nursing and Midwifery degrees in collaboration with the Oxford Schools of Nursing and Midwifery and the Oxfordshire District Health Authority's Nursing and Midwifery Service. More recently he played a key role in the Polytechnic's collaboration with Dorset House School of Occupational Therapy to develop an honours degree in Occupational Therapy.

Christopher Johns RMN, RGN, CertEd, MN

Christopher Johns is currently manager of Burford Community Hospital and Primary Care and Head of Burford Nursing Development Unit. He qualified as a nurse tutor in 1983 and worked at University College Hospital and in West Dorset before becoming senior nurse at Brackley Cottage Hospital in Oxfordshire. His current research focusses particularly on the development and support of nurses in primary nursing roles.

Anne Marie Rafferty RGN, DN, BSc, MPhil

Anne Marie Rafferty is currently lecturer in the Department of Nursing Studies, Queen's Medical Centre, University of Nottingham. She has held posts as staff nurse/research assistant, research student and nurse teacher. Her research has combined clinical and historical work. In her present post she teaches undergraduate nurses on the Bachelor of Nursing degree, students on the Health Policy and Organization MSc and research methods to post-registration nurses.

Alan Pearson PhD, RGN, ONC, DANS, MSc, FRCNA, FRCN

Alan Pearson is Professor of Nursing at Deakin University, Geelong, Australia. He has a long career in both clinical and academic work and has published widely. His current interests lie in action in nursing and therapeutic effects of nursing.

Kate Robinson PhD, BA, RGN, RHV

Kate Robinson is currently Dean of Faculty of Health Care and Social Studies, Luton College of Further Education. She took a degree in History and American Studies at Keele University and began a career in adult education before training as a nurse in Sheffield and London. She later trained as a health visitor before moving into a research post at South Bank Polytechnic and gaining a PhD in Health Studies. A post at the Open University began an interest in open and distance learning and she was the founding Director of the Distance Learning Centre at South Bank Polytechnic. She worked within the Clinical Practice Development Team, Oxford Health Authority, before moving back to the Open University.

Hugh Robinson BA, MSc, PhD, MBCS

Hugh Robinson is currently senior lecturer in computing at the Open University. His research and teaching interests centre around database technology and the construction of knowledge in computing. He has been a visiting professor at the University of Denver in Colorado, USA and has also worked in hospitals in Southampton and Tittensor, Staffordshire.

Kevin Teasdale MA(Oxon), CertEd, RMN

Kevin Teasdale trained first as a teacher, then as a psychiatric nurse. He worked in clinical areas for the elderly and in day care settings, before becoming a nurse tutor at Rauceby Hospital in South Lincolnshire. He is now Director of In Service Training for the South Lincolnshire Centre of Mid-Trent College of Nursing and Midwifery and is responsible for both continuing education in nursing and multidisciplinary training.

Barbara Vaughan MSc, RGN, DipN, DANS, RNT

Barbara Vaughan has had a distinguished career as an innovator in nursing. She was the co-author of *Models for Nursing Practice* (with Alan Pearson) and co-editor of *Managing*

Nursing Work with Moira Pillmoor. In her post as Clinical Practice Development Nurse (education) in Oxfordshire she was responsible for developing nursing theory and practice and the introduction of the lecturer practitioner role. More recently she has been involved with the establishment of a Nursing Development group in Wales in relationship to her post as Senior Lecturer in the School of Nursing Studies at the University of Wales College of Medicine. Currently, Barbara is Programme Director for Nursing Developments at the King's Fund Centre, London. A frequent contributor to the nursing press and to conferences throughout Europe, she is committed to the furtherance of nursing as an independent discipline.

Preface

If necessity was the mother of this book, the Oxford Polytechnic Department of Nursing was its godmother. During the development of the curriculum for the nursing and midwifery degrees, many elements of the programme were drawn from the basic sciences. The plans proposed that biology, sociology, chemistry, etc. would be taught, at least in part, by specialists in those areas. The students would therefore, during the first year of their studies, have to think through the place of each of the disciplines within nursing. They would have to understand that each discipline offered a different perspective on the world, developed in the main through their use of a particular method of developing knowledge. However, in our experience of such multidisciplinary courses, subject teachers often said very little about what was unique or different about their subject – rather taking for granted the issues of epistemology, that is the ways of knowing, which underpinned their thinking.

Nurses cannot take these for granted. Because they have to grapple with many basic disciplines, they need to be clear about the epistemology of each and the contribution each can make to nursing practice. And all this must form the background to their reflection on the epistemology of nursing – the ways in which nursing is known.

In order to help the students think through these issues, a short course was developed within the degree programme which would guide the students, early in their first year, in the ways of knowing that were appropriate to each basic discipline. This book was first conceived as accompanying the Oxford programme, but of course the issues which we dealt with in the context of the Oxford Polytechnic degree programme are common to all nursing programmes, whether preregistration or postregistration, diploma or degree. Nursing will always 'borrow' from basic sciences and will always have to consider the implications of that borrowing.

When faced by the daunting task of coping with a broad array of basic disciplines, students often look for and expect certainty. The display of the complex disagreements and disputes which are endemic within most sciences fills them with horror. But it is crucial that students do understand these internal disputes because they are the dynamics of the discipline; they challenge the notion that knowledge is a static wall of facts built up brick by brick and enhance the idea that knowledge is a way of looking at things, a perspective, which is not 'true' but 'good enough' until we find something better. People's ideas of what is 'good enough' differ even within a single discipline. Without this understanding the nursing students cannot appreciate that one book from a discipline may give only a very partial account of that discipline's knowledge; that books written at a certain period may contain a distinctive perspective which may have subsequently been overturned. To give you an example: although one of us (KR) is familiar with the internal discussions within sociology, she only realized some of the problems students faced in combining disciplines when sitting on an examination board and discussing useful sources of biology. Within biology, sources more than, say, ten years old were not useful and the students were discouraged from using them. Within my current teaching subject, sociology, there are many books written ten, twenty, fifty years ago which I would encourage students to read; not just as historical curiosities but as major texts for the discipline.

While we each work within our own disciplines we cannot always appreciate the problems which students have in switching between them. Sharrock (1979, p.125) describes the problem with some accuracy:

> it is not the *fact* of borrowing that poses the problem, but the uncontrolled and incautious way in which it is typically done. It is now increasingly recognized that ideas, theories and evidence take their sense and significance from the contexts in which they originate and that they are not easily extricated from those without serious distortion. Unless there is an awareness of the character of the context from which they are taken, then, and unless their detachment from that is managed with care there is every likelihood that the relevant ideas or information will be deprived of their proper or original sense, and reliability.

The first part of this book discusses the basic problems and looks at ways in which knowledge is organized. The second part offers separate accounts of some of the most important major disciplines in nursing. The third part offers some examples of how these disciplines may feed into practice. In the fourth part, some very individual perspectives on significant problems within the debate about nursing knowledge are raised. Sometimes we tend to see nursing as outside of the political, economic and technological world context, but of course all decisions are made in that context and we need to understand that broader picture.

Reference

Sharrock, W. (1979) Portraying the professional relationship, In *Health Education in Practice* (ed. D. C. Anderson), Croom Helm, London

Part One

Chapter 1

The nature of nursing knowledge

Barbara Vaughan

The idea behind this book developed when we, the editors, were faced with the dilemma of introducing students of nursing, at the very beginning of their programme, to the world of research. It raised, for us, many vital questions. Where should we begin? What constitutes nursing research? Why do students of nursing need to understand research? What type of research do they need to be introduced to in order to deepen their understanding of nursing and become safe, effective practitioners?

If research is about gaining new knowledge and insight into a given subject, then at one level these questions could be resolved very simply by launching into a series of sessions about the research process, research methods, research designs and research tools. However, as one soon learns in life, nothing is as simple as it seems at first sight. It is all very well to learn about a process but that process is meaningless unless it is put into context. It is the context of nursing research which is so complex, for it raises vital questions of what constitutes *nursing knowledge* and how nurses *acquire* that knowledge.

Thus the prime concern of this book is to begin to explore the nature of knowledge, a subject known more correctly as *espistemology*. In particular, nursing knowledge is considered, as a starting point for raising critical awareness of the knowledge which is used in practice. There is little doubt that in working through these issues more questions will be raised than answers given, as there are still huge gaps in our understanding of practice. Yet, despite this fact, there are many people who have over the years become what Benner

(1984) describes as 'expert practitioners', making decisions and taking actions which a stranger to their world may find hard to understand. How is it then that these people know what to do, what will be effective, what will work and what should be rejected? Where have they drawn their knowledge and insight from? How have they assimilated the vast range of information from the theory of both nursing and other disciplines in order to make sense of it in practice?

Some of these questions may never be answered, for it has been suggested that most people know more than they can ever put into words (Polyani, 1958) and that many actions are based on so called 'intuition'. People gain a *tacit* knowledge within themselves over time which neither they nor others can always express in words. Indeed, it is only in recent years that the value of such knowledge has been recognized and means have been sought of exploring largely uncharted 'ways of knowing' in the work of nurses and other disciplines. Being open to such ideas without rejecting more traditional approaches to enquiry can be seen as essential to the future development of the discipline of nursing.

Sources of knowledge

One view of how people gain the knowledge on which they base their assumptions and judgements suggests three prime sources, all of which should be familiar.

First, *tenacity*: that is, 'I know because it has always been like that and consequently I accept it as true' (although there is a second question here as to whether any such thing as truth can ever be attained!). This is the stuff from which many of our attitudes and current interpretations of the world around us come. For example, it was accepted as a basic truth for hundreds of years that the world was flat and the people of that time based all their assumptions on this so called 'fact'. However, we all 'know' now, as our understanding has increased, that this so-called fact has been found to be a false premise. Hence the caution in suggesting that anything is an absolute truth, for there will always be a degree of caution in a healthy, enquiring mind. Indeed, if it were not for this curiosity and challenge amongst people, the state of knowledge would never progress. One of the fundamental blocks to development is the type of mind which accepts all it currently knows without question, *tenaciously* hanging on to something which is thought to be so. We would add that this does not mean everything must be rejected which had previously been accepted as true, since no one could live in such a state. What it does suggest is that a mind which is open to new ideas is better equipped to develop.

Second, there is the knowledge which people derive from others who they perceive to be an *authority* or *expert* on the question in hand. Such knowledge may arise from the literature, from debate with experts, from role modelling or similar sources. Of course the question which has to be raised here is the legitimacy of the source. Not everything which has been written is accurate and not everything which is done is based on current understanding or good practice. A case in point would be the health care worker who, despite the wealth of knowledge suggesting that smoking is harmful to health, continues to smoke. Thus, a senior practitioner, whose behaviour could be a source of knowledge from which others could draw as a role model, may in fact exhibit unhelpful behaviour as an individual. It should be added that many experienced practitioners have indeed become experts over the years and can demonstrate more expertise than they can ever put into words. The value of the knowledge gained through well-used experience should never be underestimated, even when it cannot always be expressed succinctly. This does, of course, place considerable responsibility on the learner who, at the end of the day, must make a personal judgement about which sources of knowledge he or she will accept. However, it can also bring about an awareness of the importance of critical enquiry.

The third source of knowledge which people commonly take on board is known as '*a priori*', the knowledge which stands to reason and has been derived from logical deduction. For example, I do not have to go to Russia to know that Russia exists. There is enough evidence for its existence from other sources which my reason tells me is acceptable. Therefore I do not have to prove it for myself but will accept it as a fact. Nevertheless, my *concept* of Russia may not be entirely accurate and when I do get there I may find that I have to readjust my understanding of what it is like. Thus when I have not experienced something but deduced how it is there may be a flaw in my deduction.

Another example of this is the very wide variety of views which people hold of nurses. Most people in our society believe that nurses exist and many have a fairly strong idea of what nurses do. However, once nursing has been experienced on either the receiving or the giving end then the way in which it is understood will inevitably alter.

If we examine ourselves and ask the simple question 'How do I know?', then it can be suggested that all of us will find an element of each of these sources in our very 'knowing'. However, such knowledge does leave a great gap in our understanding, and over the years nurses have moved into a phase of seeking more certainty and understanding of what they do through the development of so-called empirical knowledge – that is, knowledge gained through empirical work by study and rigorous research. The query which we are then faced with is what areas of enquiry are legitimate for nurses to study within their work roles.

Nursing knowledge

Few people would deny that experienced practitioners of nursing draw on a wealth of knowledge when making clinical judgements. Indeed, for nearly a century the right to trade as a 'Registered Nurse' has been protected by legislation and it is only those people who have undergone an agreed programme of learning who are entitled to offer their services in this way. Implicit in this situation is the implication that there is an extensive body of knowledge required in order to be able to practise as a nurse. However, there is still the question, which vexes the minds of many concerned, of what constitutes nursing knowledge and where and how that knowledge is gained by experienced practitioners.

Carper (1978) offers a taxonomy of nursing knowledge, all parts of which she suggests come into play in any given nursing situation and her work has become almost classic in looking at nursing knowledge. She suggests that there are, in fact, four 'fundamental patterns of knowing in nursing': empirics, ethics, aesthetics and personal knowledge.

Empirics is the area of knowledge which has been gained through observation and testing of theories, taking them beyond the stage of hunches or ideas, through systematic investigation. It is based on the assumption that 'what is known is that which is accessible through the senses — that which can be seen, touched and so forth' (Chinn and Jacobs, 1987). It is in this school of thought that the majority of emphasis has been placed in trying to develop a scientific body of nursing knowledge in recent years.

Since people are the prime concern of nurses, empirical knowledge gained by many other disciplines is also of concern to them. Thus the knowledge explored by physiologists, psychologists, historians and sociologists, amongst others, acts as a backdrop to the development and understanding of nursing knowledge. This does not mean to say that such knowledge is *directly* applied in practice; rather that it becomes part of the background understanding of the practitioner which he or she can draw on and 'transform' (after Habermas, 1971) in action. As Schultz and Meleis (1988) suggest: 'They [nurses] use knowledge from other disciplines but through reflection and imagination evolve perspectives on that knowledge which are unique to nursing.'

The implication behind this statement is that in order to be able to make use of this knowledge nurses need a broad range of understanding of the different ways in which people from other disciplines undertake empirical work. For example, physiologists and sociologists use quite different approaches to enquiry (a point we shall return to), yet each has something important to offer nurses. If too much emphasis is put on one approach without respect for the others then an unbalanced picture of the person would emerge. Thus the nurses who spend all their time exploring the physiological aspects of a person at the cost of ignoring the sociological aspects would be at risk of trying to nurse a person who is only known as a physiologically functioning being, rather than as a person in a social context.

Carper (1978) and many others (Allen, 1985; Chinn and Jacobs, 1987; Meleis, 1987; Thompson, 1987) now recognize that there is much more that influences practice than empirical knowledge, and that these other 'patterns of knowing' are of equal importance.

Ethics is the notion of moral knowledge in nursing, which involves making judgements about what is right or wrong in a given situation. There is not one of us who does not have views on what is morally right or wrong, either in such major issues as abortion and euthanasia or apparently smaller issues such as to which of two patients to give the only clean sheet you have. Indeed, it has been suggested that there is a degree of morality in every decision we make (Downie and Calman, 1987), which will inevitably influence the way in which we practice, yet alone live our lives. Thus an understanding and awareness of ethics (the study of morality) can contribute significantly to practice.

It must be pointed out that morality is not necessarily made up of things which can be 'observed and tested', as in empirical science, but takes us into the realms of thought, philosophy and reflection. It raises questions such as 'Is this just or right?', which cannot always be answered directly and may cause conflict since there is often no right or wrong answer and different people hold different opinions. Attempts have been made however to draw up Codes of Conduct (United Kingdom Central Council for Nursing, 1984) based on broad ethical theories which are concerned with such things as rights and truth-telling, with the purpose of trying to guide decision-making in this complex area. Knowledge of these codes is a crucial requirement of every practitioner but the codes can only act as a guide, since morality is a personal thing within each one of us and, as such, requires a personal understanding.

Aesthetics is sometimes called the art of nursing or maybe that intuitive act which makes the expert practitioner behave in an unexpected way from time to time. It is concerned with interpreting meaning into action. Schon (1987) deepens our understanding of this when he talks of the expert sometimes being 'surprised' by a turn of events which does not 'fit the pattern' as empirics would have us expect. In this situation experts call on a whole range of past experience in order to be able to plan a new course of action which does not always seem to make sense at first sight.

What is, of course, worrying is that there is a danger of some people being caught in the net of not being able to act outside the arena of empirical knowledge because they have been schooled into thinking that this is the most important and valuable information on which to act. Again a clinical example may clarify this point. The importance of giving information to patients has been well researched and documented, and is now accepted as good practice (through empirical knowing). The new practitioner will conscientiously include this aspect of nursing when planning care and will ensure that certain information is shared, come what may. The proficient practitioner (Benner, 1984) with some years of experience will move on from this stage to also judge the time, degree and way in which the information is given. The expert practitioner, basing judgement on years of experience, may from time to time have the courage to follow 'intuition' in *not* sharing something, even though this would be the wrong act according to the text book. While drawing on empirical knowledge as a background to the decision which is made, action is based on a broad understanding of the meaning of this particular situation and the possible outcomes of any actions which are taken. Returning to the notion of knowing more than one can tell, the practitioner may have difficulty in explaining why this is so, making accountability difficult, but has the strength to act on his or her personal knowledge of the situation, and what is right for that person in that unique situation. Thus, while many of the 'acts' of nursing can be taught and basic manual skills learned fairly simply, the artistry, or the assimilation of multiple sources of knowing in order to make a decision which is right in a unique situation, requires an extensive knowledge of practice.

This takes us through to Carper's final area of knowing, that of *personal knowledge*, the knowing of self and hence the ability to trust self. Empirical knowledge from the natural sciences may offer understanding *about* oneself but Carper differentiates this from simply *knowing* self. Without this self-awareness it is difficult to see how practice can develop, since our own understanding influences everything we do. For example, to help someone who has a terminal illness and is dying without having come to terms with our own mortality would mean that a barrier would potentially exist. It is hard to understand how one can expect a patient to be honest and trusting about how he or she feels in such a situation without first being honest with self.

So many of the issues which nurses face in their everyday work, such as pain, disfigurement, loss or even less obvious things such as dealing with unpleasant smells, are hard to handle. Much can be learned from the literature in coming to understand these things yet there is a fundamental difference between knowing formally about such issues and knowing personally about them. Certainly empirical knowledge has much to offer in these areas, but if it is used alone it can lead to practice which is hidebound by a set of rules. For example, we can learn from the psychologists that denial is one means which people will use to avoid facing an undesirable reality, and such knowledge may help us to understand why people sometimes forget information they have been given in relation to their prognoses. However, recognition of the way in which we, too, may use denial cannot come from reading alone but may be gained through a degree of personal reflection. It is a form of knowing which is not always directly communicable to others but is gained over time and through experience. In using personal knowledge a new perspective comes into play as the individual perceives himself or herself to be able to adjust or modify a response, recognizing the personal aspect of the situation which is context bound in the here and now.

World views of knowledge

It has already been suggested that nurses draw on a wide range of sources of knowledge from both nursing theory and the theory developed by other disciplines. It has also been indicated that different disciplines often use different approaches to enquiry, according to the particular world view, and hence the *paradigm* they pursue. Broadly speaking there are three guiding paradigm views which have a strong influence on the way in which truth is sought, each of which is legitimate in its own right. Unfortunately, many proponents of one school of thought will reject alternative approaches, leading to a dichotomy between different fields of study. According to Hammersley and Atkinson (1983, p.3), this dichotomy is relatively new:

> where earlier, in both sociology and social psychology, qualitative and quantitative forms had generally been used side by side, often by the same researcher, there was now a tendency for distinct methodological traditions to be formed and for those legitimated by positivism to become dominant.

For nurses, who draw on knowledge from multiple sources, this could create difficulties, since each approach has something to offer. Thus it becomes important that an understanding and valuing of the knowledge gained from each of these paradigms is sought.

The natural sciences

The great majority of people who study the natural sciences, such as biology, physiology or pathology, follow a very specific research process, aiming to test out a hypothesis which they have already formulated. Thus they develop a theoretical idea and *deductively* test it out under *experimental* conditions. The essence behind this view of science arises from a school of thought called *positivism*. Its basic premise is concerned with identifying cause and effect and, in so doing, being able to identify generally applicable theories which can hold good in a multitude of circumstances. As such, some will argue that that which is not measurable cannot be scientifically explored and the use of controlled trials is the only real means of adding to our body of knowledge.

Positivism is based on certain fundamental beliefs. One is the notion of objectivity (obviously far removed from intuition!). A second is the notion of measurability. In order to be able to examine something, a means must be found of measuring it so that an idea can be formed as to whether or not it changes under certain circumstances. Furthermore, whatever tests are applied to assess the subject, they have to be repeatable in a wide range of circumstances and many times so that error of judgement can be eliminated. It is characterized by *reductionism*; that is, breaking things down into ever smaller parts in order to be able to study them, with little attention being paid to the interrelationship of the constituent parts with the whole and the way in which they interplay (for further discussion, see Hammersley and Atkinson, 1983)

Thus, for example, someone's degree of stress in a particular situation can be assessed either through physiological measurements, such as levels of catecholamines in the blood (a very legitimate, well-proven measurement), or through self-report or the use of prevalidated psychological tests (which may be less well proven but nevertheless acceptable). In this way a relationship can be sought between a named nursing intervention and the degree of stress in a patient. This approach to enquiry is the one which is most commonly used in the so-called scientific world (including medicine) and is definitely the one which gains most credence either when seeking a research grant or ethical approval. Certainly it is an approach which is most widely understood by disciplines other than our own.

It must be emphasized at this stage that the degree of knowledge which has been gained through this approach is vast, and its importance should never be underestimated. However, it is also worth pointing out that it does have major limitations. There are some areas of knowing which do not lend themselves readily to measurement in this way, since they cannot always be reduced to measurable items. This is certainly the case with many aspects of nursing. Furthermore, one also has to question whether anyone can ever be truly objective and deny a personal perspective of the world we live in.

Again, an example may make this point clearer. Suppose there was an interest in trying to find out if a certain dressing was more effective in aiding healing of a leg ulcer than its counterpart. In a very straightforward way a clinical trial could be undertaken to compare the effectiveness of the two dressings. Further, it would be possible to match the sample of patients used for any other factors which might be relevant, such as age, respiratory and circulatory function and so forth. In this way a vast amount of material could be gained to provide knowledge of this situation and maybe validate a theory related to the potential value of a particular dressing.

Within the positivist framework such an approach would be entirely justified and, indeed, this would be a very useful source of information on which to base a clinical judgement in the future. However, there is a fundamental weakness in this approach to science, based on the principle that while it may be possible to prove something to be false, in this instance that one dressing appears to be no better than the other, it is not possible to prove *absolutely* that anything is completely true. It can only be suggested that there is high *probability* that it is true according to the information which has been gathered to date. This 'flaw in the system' arises from two basic premises. First, in 'manipulating and controlling' the situation, as one must in experimental conditions, reality may be altered. Thus findings would only be true if the experimental conditions were also repeated. Second, in setting up the trial in the first place the investigator may have forgotten to control for 'factor X', not intentionally but because its relevance to the situation being tested was not recognized or it was outside the personal reference system of the investigator. Returning to the example given above, it may be that there is an association between 'hope' (a difficult thing to quantify) and the healing of leg ulcers. If hope is not seen as measurable and hence easily *quantified* then it would not come into the 'thinking' of the positivist investigator, particularly as it does not fit a basic assumption of the positivist that everything can be reduced to measurable factors. However, it could be that this was just the thing which skewed the results and gave what could be a false picture.

The example given here is simplistic but this might not always be the case. For instance, think back to the thalidomide tragedy (a well-tested drug which had been accepted by our scientific control methods as safe): 'factor X', in this instance the effect the drug might have on a fetus, was not considered and the results were tragic.

Thus while positivism has a role to play, it also has drawbacks. One of these drawbacks is that it stands back from the world it examines, and in looking at it objectively it may not recognize the views or critical factors of those within that world. This takes us on to another form of enquiry, the one which may just help us to identify factor X.

Naturalism

In response to the concerns which some people have about the positivist world view an alternative school of thought has developed, most commonly known as *naturalism*. Those who follow this school of thought suggest that 'as far as possible the world should be studied in its "natural" state, undisturbed by the researcher' (Hammersley and Atkinson, 1983, p.6). They suggest that it is not always possible to understand everything in a 'cause and effect' relationship, since different things take on different meanings to people in different circumstances. Thus it is no good setting up a health education programme for a specific group of people unless there is an understanding of what constitutes good health in *their* eyes, since the programme will be meaningless if their view of good health differs from that of those offering the programme. In many ways this matches the holistic philosophy which underlies modern nursing practice, since, borrowing words from Virginia Henderson (1966), it entails getting inside someone's skin to try to see the world as they view it. In this way many of the factors which you or I as health care workers may not have considered relevant can come to light. For example, in one small study relating to community care for those families who have a child with mental handicap in their midst, what became quite clear was that 'community care' is a misnomer and it is 'family care' which happens in reality, with quite severe perceived isolation from the community. Now, whether or not this can be seen to be happening through measurable means, i.e. a reduced number of social contacts and so forth, the important factor from a study of this kind is that this is how the *recipients* of the service perceive reality and thus their perceived need for help. There are very obvious implications for the redressing of the services provided in such work as either use of or compliance with a service is likely to be minimal if it does not match the need felt.

This *interpretative* view of the world moves away from seeing the research subjects as passive objects to be studied from a distance, to a shared experience, the 'us' experience, where the researcher and the subject work together to deepen understanding. Rather than testing hypotheses deductively in experimental conditions, the situation is explored as it *is* and an attempt is made to interpret its meaning, as it is seen by the people who are participating in that particular scene. In this way greater insight can be gained of the 'real world'.

Theories are not usually tested, as in the positivist approach, but *may* be formulated from the insight gained through such study. There are a multitude of ways in which this work can be realized, looking at such approaches as phenomenology (trying to identify/clarify the meaning of phenomena), ethnography (story-telling from the recipient's point of view), hermeneutics (looking at the meaning of language in context), and so forth. The essential essence is to try and deepen our shared understanding of the world, which in turn may influence our actions. Thus, instead of looking for cause and effect, as in positivism, meanings and understanding are sought. This method also has limitations as well as values since it would never be possible to study a total picture of a given phenomenon, culture or situation and the methods of enquiry may themselves still give a degree of distortion. Nevertheless it offers an alternative approach which can help to build a picture of reality.

Critical social theory

Having briefly outlined the notions of positivism and naturalism, which both have a major contribution to make to nursing knowledge, a third view is what has been called *critical social theory*. In recent years the positivist and naturalist schools of thought have been challenged, primarily by the so-called Frankfurt school of neomarxist thinking. Habermas (1971) puts forward the notion that the 'empirico-analytical' approach to understanding only provides one important perspective of knowledge which gives rise to an ability to manipulate the environment in order to achieve predefined ends. Alongside this he acknowledges the place of the 'interpretative' school of thought, where understanding is based on an interpretation of social interactions.

However, Habermas and others of this school (e.g. Giroux, 1983) add a third dimension to these two sources of knowledge: they have called it the 'critical paradigm', which is primarily concerned with *emancipation of self*. They argue that, rather than directly adding to total world knowledge, critical theory is concerned with the human ability to act rationally, to make decisions in the light of available knowledge, to gain a greater understanding of self. It is primarily concerned with *controlling* the knowledge gained through technical and interpretative enquiry, using actions to realize personal, social and professional goals.

Critical science arises out of the notion that theory is embedded in practice but that 'actual knowledge is always limited in some sense by the sociohistorical context in which it arises' (Allen, 1985). Thus each person is limited by his or her social and historical background, some groups being more powerful than others in controlling what is currently happening. Deeper understanding of the things which place limitations on our own actions can lead to emancipation and *praxis* (or change through action), in line with the work of Friere (1972). By these means people may gain understanding of self, becoming autonomous agents of change through their own actions. In this way change grows creatively from reflection on action rather than being limited to the application of theory deductively. Critical theory is explored through *action research*, which acknowledges the value and place of both technical and interpretative theory but intentionally seeks change through reflection on action (Carr and Kemmis, 1984).

So this final area of research lies very much on the participative end of a continuum of sources of so-called legitimate knowledge. It is an area still largely unexplored in nursing but may well have something to offer which can complement other approaches to enquiry and enhance the contribution which nurses can offer in the health care arena. The methodology of this area is still in its infancy but according to Chin and Jacobs (1987) the data can only be validated by the person concerned because it is so personal. However, what it does do is challenge, and in some instances *transform* or alter traditional theory and place value on discovery through action, i.e. the discovery of the practitioner immersed in the situation alongside that of either the participant observer or the objective scientist.

There is, of course, a danger in suggesting that the nursing work force is emancipated in this way. Control is gone and some will take liberty, using it as an excuse for not bothering to explore what is known from other sources of knowledge. It is suggested here that this is *not* what emancipation is about. It is the confidence to awaken a critical view of the world, alongside a confidence to trust your own judgement in balance with the formal espoused theory. It entails respect for self, alongside respect for the contributions of others. If this is not the stance taken then the oppressed can become the oppressor. Maybe this is particularly important in nursing, where nurses as a group have been oppressed for a multitude of reasons, such as gender issues, their perceived role in society and their subservient relationship to medicine. The last thing we want is a group of nurses who presume their form of knowing is best and in so doing try to oppress others, mainly by decrying the importance of the contribution of medicine and, even more importantly, the vast self-knowledge that patients already have. What we do want is a people who are sufficiently emancipated to stand up in a multidisciplinary group and value the contribution they have to make to the total health care picture (for further discussion, see Smythe, 1986).

Knowledge of practice

Schon (1983) suggests that lack of recognition of the so-called 'intuitive knowledge' of practice has been accentuated over the years with the place which has been given by society to more traditional theory; ideas which are supported by Benner and Wrubel (1989). It is often this formal theory which is used as the basis of education in practice disciplines. Thus, very often, what is taught does not reflect the form of knowledge which is used by expert practitioners, but the knowledge of practice is not valued nor is it readily available or accessible through others. It can, however, develop through self-growth and reflection on actions in reality, which may in turn lead to a challenge to some aspects of positivist or interpretative theory, perpetually challenging the status quo and leading to change.

In her earlier work, Benner (1984) supports these ideas as she speaks of the way in which expert practitioners learn their skills. She is critical of the continuous movement of students from one setting to another, suggesting that they never have time to get beyond the stage of novice in acquiring rule-led skills. Her premise acknowledges the complex developmental stages through which practitioners progress in order to gain expert status. If insufficient time is allowed for people to move beyond the stage of learning a series of actions to be applied in a given situation, they cannot either understand through observation how others make decisions nor recognize the complex contextual cues which free them from rule-bound actions to become creative practitioners themselves.

It can be suggested that an understanding of the nature of nursing knowledge is a prerequisite to the development of an understanding of nursing research. Without this insight there is a danger that attention will be focused on inappropriate areas of enquiry and the knowledge gained from other sources will either go unrecognized or be misused and applied in a rule-bound way. As Meleis (1987) suggests:

> we should focus our investigations on the domain of nursing, develop gender sensitive knowledge, use global approaches to knowledge development and use multiple approaches to conceptualize and investigate phenomena.

This offers a challenge to all those who are concerned with the future development of nursing knowledge as they need to gain insight and respect for a multitude of perspectives on knowledge. However, it also offers the opportunity to find new and creative ways of developing methods and approaches which will enhance our understanding of nursing practice.

Conclusion

This chapter has set out to raise an awareness of the different approaches which can be taken in exploring the world we live in. Knowledge can be gained from many different sources, each of which has something to offer in our total understanding or 'knowing' and it is important that recognition, understanding and respect are gained for all these schools of thought.

The following chapters are contributed from people working in many different disciplines, offering insight into the predominant way in which they undertake enquiry. By the very nature of their different schools of thought the chapters vary in style and approach, which can be seen as a reflection of the varying views and opinions which they hold. This is an

18   Knowledge for Nursing Practice

intentional act since to edit them in such a way as to make
them all 'similar' would be against the underlying purpose of
this book and would deny their very individual approaches. It
is hoped that the complementary way in which they can all
contribute to nursing knowledge will become apparent.

References

Allen, D. (1985) Nursing research and social control: alternative
    models of science that emphasize understanding and emancipa-
    tion. *Image – The Journal of Nursing Scholarship*, 17(2), 58–64
Benner, P. (1984) *From Novice to Expert; Excellence and Power in
    Clinical Nursing Practice*, Addison-Wesley, Menlo Park CA
Benner, P. and Wrubel, J. (1989) *The Primacy of Caring*, Addison-
    Wesley, Menlo Park CA
Carper, B. (1978) Fundamental patterns of knowing in nursing.
    Advances in Nursing Science, 1(1), 13–23
Carr, W. and Kemmis, S. (1984) *Becoming Critical: Knowing Through
    Action Research*, Deakin University Press, Victoria
Chinn, P. and Jacobs, M. (1987) *Theory and Nursing: A Systematic
    Approach*, Mosby, St Louis
Downie, R.S. and Calman, K.C. (1987) *Healthy Respect: Ethics in
    Health Care*, Faber and Faber, London
Friere, P. (1972) *Pedagogy of the Oppressed*, Penguin, Harmonds-
    worth, UK
Giroux, H. (1983) *Critical Theory and Educational Practice*, Deakin
    University Press, Victoria
Habermas, J. (1971) *Knowledge and Human Interests* (translated by J.
    Shapiro), Beacon, Boston MA
Hammersley, M. and Atkinson, P. (1983) *Ethnography: Principles in
    Practice*, University Press, Cambridge
Henderson, V. (1966) *The Nature of Nursing*, Collier MacMillan,
    London
Meleis, A. (1987) Revisions in knowledge development: a passion for
    substance. *Scholarly Enquiry for Nursing Practice – An International
    Journal*, 1(1), 5–19
Polyani, M. (1958) *Personal Knowledge: Towards a Postcritical Philo-
    sophy*, Harper Torchbooks, New York
Schon, D. (1983) *The Reflective Practitioner – How Professionals Think
    in Action*, Temple Smith, London
Schon, D. (1987) *Educating the Reflective Practitioner*, Jossey-Bass,
    Oxford
Schultz, P. and Meleis, A. (1988) Nursing epistemology: traditions,
    insights, questions. *Image – Journal of Nursing Scholarship*, 20(4),
    217–221
Smythe, W.J. (1986) *Reflection in Action*, Deakin University Press,
    Victoria

Thompson, J. (1987) Critical scholarship: the critique of domination in nursing. *Advances in Nursing Science*, **10(1)**, 27–38

United Kingdom Central Council for Nursing, Midwifery and Health Visiting (1984) *The Code of Professional Conduct for Nurses, Midwives and Health Visitors*, UKCC, London

Part Two
Sources of Knowledge

Each of the following chapters is concerned with one academic discipline. The concept of a discipline is hard to define clearly but it refers to an organizational framework within which knowledge is produced and passed on. The *Shorter Oxford English Dictionary* (1980) defines it as 'A branch of instruction; a department of knowledge'. The idea of compartmentalizing knowledge in this way is a fundamental 'given' of our higher educational system, although it had been increasingly abandoned within the school system until the advent of the national curriculum. However, it is important to say that the traditional compartments, which appear here, are not fixed and immutable but can and do change. Boundaries within and between disciplines are continually evolving. However, we have retained these discipline descriptions here because they are well used and understood within nursing. They all contribute substantially to the new curricula for nurse education. They do not, however, constitute a complete list of the disciplines which could or should contribute to nurse education. Economics is perhaps the most notable omission, but we should also like to see the inclusion of the arts, particularly literature, and social geography, which is the study of the relationship between social organization and space (for example, see Gregory and Urry, 1985). However, nursing does not yet draw substantially on these disciplines; hopefully a future edition could include them.

There is a current debate within nursing about who should teach these basic disciplines. We have taken a pragmatic view. Some of the contributors are nurses who have an interest in another academic area, others are academics in basic disciplines who have developed an interest in nursing. Their brief as writers was to take a critical look at their discipline, to discuss the ways in which enquiry was undertaken within it, and to highlight some of the internal controversies and complexities. Obviously there has not been space for an exhaustive overview of each discipline, and those needing a detailed description will find references to useful textbooks within each chapter. Here, we have been more interested in emphasizing the 'cutting edge' of the discipline: the places where there is debate and conflict about the very nature of the subject as well as the knowledge base produced.

The chapters vary in style and approach and we have encouraged this diversity. The way in which a subject is talked about is a reflection of the varying views and opinions within the subject. To impose uniformity would be to deny some of the 'specialness' of each subject's perspective and would therefore defeat one of the purposes of this book.

There are many themes and messages contained in the chapters of Part Two and, depending on your own interests and experience, you will doubtless focus on some more than others. However, we would like to draw your attention to some of the messages which seem to us to appear and re-appear throughout the chapters.

First, we return to the issue raised in Part One: that knowledge cannot be 'mined' from basic disciplines in any simple fashion. The production of knowledge resides in a particular time and space and must be connected to the context in which it is produced. Second, there is by no means agreement within any discipline about the best way to go about producing knowledge. 'How do we know things to be true?' is still a live question; perhaps Chapter 6 best exemplifies this.

But while there is a general awareness that the social sciences are engaged in vigorous internal debate it is perhaps less well known that a relatively 'hard' science such as biology is also subject to internal conflict and controversy. Chapter 3 is a useful antidote to those who wish to cling to the idea that the basic academic disciplines can bring us certainty. For it is clear from all these chapters that nothing is certain, nothing fixed. And that brings us to perhaps the most important theme which runs through all the chapters: the excitement and sheer fun of the discussions about knowledge. To make sense of our world remains the most exciting journey of all, and perhaps nurses need to appreciate that research within basic sciences is not just done so that it can be applied by others to current practical problems, but also because scientists are people who want to make sense of the world as an end in itself. As Malraux says:

> The greatest mystery is not that we have been flung at random among the profusion of the earth and the galaxy of the stars, but that in this prison we can fashion images of ourselves sufficiently powerful to deny our nothingness.

References

Gregory, D. and Urry, J. (eds) (1985) *Social Relations and Spatial Structures*, Macmillan Education, Basingstoke

Shorter Oxford English Dictionary (1980) University Press, Oxford

Chapter 2

Historical perspectives

Anne Marie Rafferty

As with nursing, 'history' may be defined in terms of its subject matter or its methods. It may also have multiple objectives, being concerned with recovering and ordering aspects of the past as well as evaluating the significance of those events in the light of contemporary concerns. This chapter is designed to give a brief introduction to some of the different approaches that have been taken to the writing of nursing history. It is not an exhaustive exploration of the subject but aims to give some idea of what you can expect to find on the historical agenda in nursing.

First, it is useful to consider what historians have perceived as their role and function in general, and in nursing in particular. This in itself is a matter for debate, but let us look first of all at the statements from two different sources. The historian David Cannadine (1987) in a viewpoint article on the past, present and future prospects for the study of British history, commented:

> Historians are the mediators between the past and the present ... we are in being and in business to understand people and events in time and to communicate that understanding to a wider audience ... But we are constrained in these endeavours, not only by the limitations of the historical evidence and individual imagination but also by those contemporary pre-occupations which in one way or another, invariably affect us all, and thus in part influence the kind of history we write. (p. 171)

Compare this statement with that of a co-author (Sarnecky, 1990, p.2) of a nursing research journal article:

greater attention to the practice of historiography promises to profit the discipline of nursing. It will not only enhance professional unity and integrity, but also embellish the artistic side of disciplinary practice, enabling nurses to view humanity more fully from a holistic perspective. It will foster the development of nursing knowledge, show us the error of our ways, act as a source of professional pride, and also provide a spiritual sense of inspiration, thereby encouraging nursing professionals to strive to achieve inconceivable heights.

What differences do you notice in the orientations and objectives of the two statements? Whilst the first author invites his audience to be alert to the potential impact of our contemporary concerns on the writing of history, the second seems to advocate the use of history for certain professional, ideological and didactic ends.

Throughout this chapter we shall look at how both these approaches have informed research and writing in the history of nursing.

In the beginning

When examining any piece of evidence or writing it is important, where possible, to consider the context and reasons for which it was produced or written. The sources of evidence upon which the historian may draw include documents or written evidence, oral sources, film, photographs, art or architecture. One of the earliest textbooks on nursing history was written by Sarah Tooley who, although not herself a nurse, was none the less sympathetic to nursing reform (Tooley, 1906). She wrote this historical survey after having completed a biography of Florence Nightingale (Tooley, 1903). The textbook seems to have been inspired by a desire to claim a place for nursing in the 'civilizing mission' of the British Empire and to help restore faith in Britain's fading imperial fortunes. The 'missionary' export of British nurses and nursing to various parts of the Empire is applauded and condoned. The author describes her reasons for writing the book in florid terms (Tooley, 1906, Preface):

The rise and spread of trained nursing is one of the most remarkable developments of the last half of the nineteenth century. It is a matter for national pride that Great Britain has been the cradle of this beneficent movement. No other country can show a like record, and though America has a highly organized and efficient system of training, it modelled its early training schools on that of St Thomas' Hospital. The name of Florence Nightingale has been wafted across the Atlantic, and when the brave daughters of America volunteered to go out and nurse 'the boys' during the civil war they were inspired by the example of the heroine of the Crimea.

Many of the early nursing histories were written by nurse reformers and their supporters (Nutting and Dock, 1907–1912; Dock and Stewart, 1920; Breay and Bedford Fenwick, 1928). Indeed, it can be argued that such accounts form an intrinsic part of, or extension of, their reform campaigns. Overall their general tone tends to be congratulatory, often extolling the pioneering efforts of nurse leaders who struggled heroically to further 'the cause' in the face of great adversity. An example of this 'lone crusader' syndrome is represented by the extract (Dock and Stewart, 1920, p.366) below:

On the whole, nurses have every reason to be proud. The great nursing leaders, whose example we want to keep always before us, were first of all great nurses, but with all their tenderness and devotion, they were vigorous, forceful, persistent, capable men and women, with clear vision and judgment, and with fearless courage.

The statement above typifies the eulogistic quality of much early writing in the history of nursing. But it is not only the context, tone and style of the account which is important, the starting point and standpoint of the discourse may also be revealing. It is significant, but not surprising perhaps, given the histories and objectives of the authors themselves, that much of the early history of nursing was written from the point of view of the nursing leadership. It is often taken for granted in such accounts that the interests of the leadership are synonymous with those of the rank and file. The possibility of inconsistency or tension between the interests of the leadership and the rank and file is rarely considered or may not even have entered the consciousness of the authors. Leaders tend to be represented positively as activists, heroic campaigners, beleaguered reformers and champions of noble causes. Whilst this approach may be sustainable on the strength of some of the evidence, it also has a number of consequences for the writing of nursing history. First, it tends to represent an image of the professional leadership as the pilot of change and controller of its own destiny. This strategy promotes an 'internalist' view of history: that is, one written from and controlled by 'insiders' which takes little account of the impact of wider social forces upon the occupation. This paints only a partial picture of events and may distort the complex interplay of forces shaping change. By so doing, it may obscure rather than clarify the factors which inhibit nurses from taking command of their own destiny. Another feature of 'internalist' accounts is that they tend to be uncritical and oriented towards sustaining a positive image of the leadership. Whilst such a tendency may be explained by the style, status, even individualism of the authors themselves, it under-represents the options available in determining decision-making strategies.

The 'progress' of politics: early histories of nursing

But what other factors have shaped the early accounts of nursing history? As you will have noticed from the excerpts above, political interests often have a powerful effect upon the substance of accounts. The monumental four-volume history by Adelaide Nutting and Lavinia Dock, for example, was published at a time when the questions of nurses' registration and women's suffrage were high on the nursing political agenda (Nutting and Dock, 1907–1912). For some, the two were inextricably linked. Mrs Bedford Fenwick, an ardent proregistrationist suffragist and leading nurse reformer, declared the nurse question was the woman question (Baly, 1986, p.295). (For brief biographical details of Mrs Bedford Fenwick see Dingwall, Rafferty and Webster, 1988, pp.78–79). Lavinia Dock was a close colleague of Mrs Bedford Fenwick and shared many of her views on the position of women as nurses and Mrs Bedford Fenwick's concern for professionalism. Miss Dock was also a co-founder, with Mrs Bedford Fenwick, of the International Council of Nurses, an organization dedicated to the promotion of educational reform, professional organization and international cooperation in nursing. Miss Dock disseminated her views on nursing reform to a British readership through the *British Journal of Nursing*, which Mrs Bedford Fenwick bought and edited from 1899, and Mrs Bedford Fenwick's views were referred to in papers published by Miss Dock in the *American Journal of Nursing*. Thus, from the earliest days of nursing journalism, ideas, opinions and views have been exchanged between British and American nurses across the Atlantic.

In the first history of the International Council of Nurses, written by two prominent members of the early organization, Margaret Breay (Honorary Secretary) and Mrs Bedford Fenwick (President), the objectives of the organization were stated as follows:

> Nurses, above all other things at present, require to be united. The value of their work to the sick is acknowledged at the present day by the government of this and of all other civilized countries, but it depends upon nurses individually and collectively to make their work of the utmost usefulness to the sick, and this can only be accomplished if their education is based on such broad lines that the term trained nurse shall be equivalent to that of a person who has received such an efficient training and has proved to be also so trustworthy that the responsible duties which she must undertake may be performed to the utmost benefit of those entrusted to her charge. To secure these results two things are essential; that there should be recognized systems of nursing education and control over the nursing profession. The experience of the past has proved that these results can never be obtained by any profession unless it is united in its demands for the necessary reform and by union alone can the necessary strength be obtained. I venture to contend that the work of nursing is one of every land without distinction of class or degree or nationality. If the poet's dream of a brotherhood of man is ever to be fulfilled, surely a sisterhood of nurses is an international idea, and one to which the women of all nations, therefore could be asked and expected to join (Breay and Bedford Fenwick, 1928–1929, pp.217–218).

It is this particular blend of internationalism, suffragism and registrationism which characterizes the Nutting and Dock volumes and informed the nature of their professional models of nursing. These accounts are particularly important since they seemed to have provided the stylistic template for later textbooks (Pavey, 1938; Seymour, 1954). Characteristic of these accounts is that they cover a vast terrain in time and space at great speed. Depth in some cases is sacrificed to breadth, and few are the product of extensive original re-search. They are none the less important records of contem-porary opinion and valuable mirrors of and guides to the political climate in which they were produced.

The politics of 'progress'

A further feature of the early histories of nursing is their tendency towards representing the historical process as a linear development towards an increasing and, by implication, inevitable perfectability. This 'progress-oriented' view is also known as the 'Whig' interpretation of history, which had its origins in the nineteenth century view of British history as the development of liberty, parliamentary rule and religious toleration common in 'Whig' intellectual circles (Wilson and Ashplant, 1988). The word 'progress' is so much a taken-for-granted part of our perceptions and vocabulary that it is difficult to imagine it as a concept whose validity may be only relevant to a part of humanity for part of the time, or indeed that it is a notion which itself has only a relatively recent history (Pollard, 1968, p.vi). A belief in 'progress' suggests that, on the basis of history, a pattern of law-like regularities can be discerned, making it possible to engage in some form of scientific prediction of the future. It also involves the assump-tion that the direction of change is invariably from a less towards a more favourable state of affairs. It is important to recognize that evaluations of 'progress' involve value judge-ments on the part of those defining the situation and that it is therefore a concept with multiple meanings. For example, the present Government might consider 'progress' in community care as more elderly being cared for in their homes in the face of reductions in expenditure on the personal, health and social services for the elderly. However, the elderly themselves, and possibly those caring for them in their homes, may not perceive the reduction or withdrawal of formal support ser-vices as 'progress'. But what are the implications and conse-quences of a 'progress-oriented' approach to the writing of nursing history?

First it might be useful to speculate on the reasons why the Whig approach has such an appeal for nurse historians, and indeed their audience. History as 'progress' may have an important psychological and morale-boosting effect, but al-though its intentions may be sound, its validity may be questioned. History can also be used to perform a range of pedagogical functions as a source of inspiration and socialization to newcomers to the occupation. The differential representation of Florence Nightingale's career to different audiences of student nurses illustrates the multiple social and ideological functions a symbolic character such as Miss Nightingale might serve (Whittaker and Olesen, 1974). But by emphasizing the 'success' stories, such history overshadows and prejudges the 'failures'. This may deny the audience the opportunity of arriving at an independent judgement of the evidence. Furthermore, this mode of representation may involve selection and a series of value judgements which seriously bias the account in favour of one point of view rather than another. It also supports what might be called the 'internal dynamic' theory of change, in which change is portrayed as originating from within and controlled by the occupation. As a consequence it may tacitly ignore those factors which inhibit and obstruct change and play down the importance of the conservative forces which provide for stability and continuity rather than change. A comprehensive understanding of the multiplicity of factors which make and break change is essential to a full understanding of events.

The critical context

The second feature of this view of history as 'progress' is that it tends to be 'nurse oriented' and highly individualistic. It fails, however, to take account of the complex political and social context in which nurses and nursing work subsists. The prominence given to a select few diminishes rather than enhances opportunities for understanding the roles of 'communities', pressure groups and collective action in managing social change. Furthermore, the view of the past as an imperfect version of the present, unfolding in a neat sequence towards infinite improvement, is strained when considered in the context of nurses' social and power relations with doctors, or their capacity to determine their own conditions of service. What may be 'progress' for one group may not imply improvement for another. Feminist historians in particular have challenged some of the concepts, analyses and periodizations used in mainstream history as not necessarily applying equally to men and women. Thus Kelly-Gadol questions whether women had a 'renaissance' and Lewis challenges the view of expansion in employment opportunities for women as being one of uninterrupted and steady progression towards sexual equality (Kelly-Gadol, 1977; Lewis, 1984, p.222).

Models of history: primate as 'primary' nursing

But what kinds of explanatory models have been used by nurse historians to organize their accounts and where did they come from? Nutting and Dock begin their first volume with an account of 'First aid in the animals' to illustrate what they claim is the instinctual basis of caring behaviour and altruism. Drawing upon the work of a Russian zoologist, Kropotkin, Nutting and Dock (1907, p.6) use the ethological basis of caring behaviour to endorse a nativist theory of caring behaviour, arguing:

> The species which have survived the most extensively and are the most capable of survival, and the theory that competition is the predominating law of life, and the 'struggle' for the means of existence ... of every man against all other men, 'a law of Nature' ... lacked confirmation from direct observation.

Kropotkin rejected Darwin's thesis that it was competition between species which determined the survival of the fittest. Drawing upon his own observations across the great geographical expanses of Russia, he claimed to find no evidence of population pressure or 'struggle for existence' in the animal world. Rather, he suggested the opposite occurred: that the more 'successful' species were those who cooperated with each other (Kropotkin, 1902). That Nutting and Dock took the animal kingdom as their starting point suggests a commitment to analogizing the biological and social worlds. This was not an unusual explanatory device to use. Appeals to what appears to be 'natural' have been and will continue to be made to support social and political programmes of various descriptions. In some senses Nutting and Dock can be considered critics of Darwin, as Karl Marx was some decades earlier when he railed against Darwin for representing the natural world as one of free competition (Thomas, 1983, p.90). The exercise of unfettered and fierce competition seemed to Marx to suggest a determinism, and fatalism in which the weak would perish and the strong continue to flourish was anathema to Marx and undermined the reforms fought and struggled for by Miss Nutting and Miss Dock. The authors were writing at a time when evolutionary biology was a subject of heated debate in educated circles. Darwin had a profound effect upon how time and the process of change were perceived by historians, scientists and writers of fiction (Morton, 1984).

Knowledge as interests

The 'new' evolutionary ideology lent scientific legitimation to a multitude of 'causes', including that of nursing. The need to locate 'nursing' in a respectable intellectual tradition may be considered part of a status-sanctioning strategy organized by a new and emerging social group. Thus 'knowledge', and in this case historical knowledge, was used to sustain claims to status. Suggesting an association between a universal and inborn characteristic such as 'caring' and the activities of a community of workers may provide a useful technique to raise the standing of that group in the public's estimation.

An additional strategy might consist in identifying the roots of an occupation's work in a reputable yet remote culture such as classical antiquity. The Nutting and Dock history takes both the scientific and ethological as well as the human and classical civilizations as their starting points. This also suggests a broad interpretation of nursing work is being taken, rather than one which focuses on the activity as paid employment and the preserve of those officially licensed to practise. The association of the origins of an occupation with antiquity and classical learning may also reflect a concern to claim a noble and prestigious pedigree for the occupation and its work. The link between classical learning and elite traditions, such as the public school system, have been analysed in the sociology of education and have been used as one means of rationing social privileges, such as access to certain kinds of employment and social positions (Campbell, 1970, pp.249–264). Bolgar (1954, p.1) has argued that during the Edwardian period, for example, the student of Greats could still have reason to believe he (note the gender identification) possessed the magic key to unlock the kingdoms of the world. In 1965, Eton had 37 masters teaching classics, 19 science, 19 mathematics and 19 other languages including English (Campbell, 1970, p.251). Groups keen to secure certain privileges may adopt the same traditions advocated by those perceived as already having achieved success. This may be particularly important in nursing, where the reality of the work may be at variance with lofty ideals claimed as inspiring it.

Historiography of nursing and medicine

The context in which history is written may be as important as the substance of the account. The prosuffragist stance of Dock and Stewart's work is evident from the manner in which nursing politics are situated within the wider context of the women's movement. This is most forcibly illustrated in Dock and Stewart's shorter single volume on the history of nursing (Dock and Stewart, 1920, p.347):

> It is, however, ... plain, that many of the difficulties which nurses have faced in the past, have been due to the fact that most of them were women, labouring under hereditary handicaps, which we have just recently begun to remove. In a paper on the 'Evolution of the Trained Nurse', Mrs Fenwick closes with the statement: 'The evolution of the trained nurse in the future depends on the evolution of woman'. We might apply this to the whole history of nursing and say that the status of nursing in all countries and at all times, has depended, not entirely, but to a very large extent on the status of women and on the degree of freedom which they have enjoyed ... With political enfranchisement there is more hope that in our own and other countries, women may be freed from many of their ancient disabilities and may be able to give their strength more freely and fully to nursing and to other branches of public service.

The line of argument and interpretive framework of accounts such as this is clear: what is being promoted here is a professional model of nursing, one in which reformers sought recognition for nursing as an independent profession from medicine. Therefore, throughout the account an attempt is made to illustrate the differential development of the two (Dock and Stewart, 1920, p.337):

> It is sometimes argued that because nursing is so closely identified with the practice of medicine, it cannot be given an independent professional status, but must be considered as a kind of 'satellite' of medicine. A very brief review of the historical relations of nursing and medicine will show that nursing is not an outgrowth of medicine, but has had an independent development for many hundreds of years.

Miss Dock was, according to Miss Stewart, the more outspoken and committed feminist of this historical collaboration (Christy, 1971, p.290). Having described the alleged independent 'curve' of development for medicine and nursing, the authors (Dock and Stewart, 1920, p.341) then invoke a 'modern', profeminist version of the familiar domestic relationship to describe their view of what the social relations between nurses and doctors should be:

> Nursing is sometimes called the 'official wife' of medicine but it is a self sustaining, not a dependent relationship, that of the modern helpmate or partner, not in the old subordinate relationship of household drudge or handmaid, that we find the truest conception of the nurse's place in the family of medicine.

History can also be used to legitimate the pursuit of autonomy by nurses. Yet in terms of the organization and style of nursing history texts, these bear a very close resemblance to those in medicine. Perhaps this represents another case of nursing following the example of medicine, but the organizational format may also be one common to professional histories of the period. None the less, there is a paradox involved in the use of history by nurses to support claims to independence from medicine, whilst using medical history as a framework for organizing such accounts. Striking similarities in the starting points and organization of medical and nursing history textbooks would strongly suggest that nursing historiography has mirrored medical historiography (Garrison, 1929). Both tend to begin their accounts with the ancient world and both utilize a grand survey approach, traversing large expanses of time and space. Just as medical history has traditionally been concerned with the history of the élite institutions, practitioners and scientific innovation, nursing history has tended to focus on leaders from prestigious institutions and educational reform. Unlike medical history, which can boast a healthy stock of scientific heroes, the supply of nursing heroines seems somewhat meagre by comparison. The character and charisma of Florence Nightingale has tended to overshadow the claims of any other candidates to heroic treatment (Whittaker and Olson, 1964). But this qualitative advantage is no compensation for the quantitative dearth of nurses who have attained public recognition and respect. The enduring success of Miss Nightingale as the dominant emblematic character in nursing can be regarded as something of a mixed blessing. For, whilst the occupation may have benefited from status gains through association with Miss Nightingale, the investment of so much symbolic significance in one person may ultimately restrict the political space within which nurses perceive they can manoeuvre. The survival of Miss Nightingale, therefore, as a strong representational character may have significant political consequences for nurses which are not necessarily empowering. It indicates the need for more searching and critical studies of the gendered nature of nursing history and its implications for political explanation and understanding.

Recent historiography of nursing

As previously mentioned, the format of the early Nutting and Dock volumes served as a blueprint for later textbooks such as those of Agnes Pavey (1938) and Lucy Seymour (1954). The interpretive framework used by later authors is also similar insofar as they tend to perpetuate the proreformist line. Until recently, therefore, nursing history textbooks have provided opportunities for endorsing the ambitions of the leadership. The first breakthrough work which examined nursing history from a standpoint which was not dominated by that of the leadership, was that of Brian Abel-Smith (1960). Interestingly, this 'deviant' work originated as an outgrowth from the author's research into the history of hospitals and, therefore, in some sense, developed by chance (Abel-Smith, 1964). It does focus on the dominant role of the hospital in the historiography as well as the professionalization of nursing. Drawing for the first time on a range of official and semiofficial reports, papers and journal articles, Abel-Smith concentrated on the 'politics' of general nursing from 1800 to 1951, set within the context of changing patterns of medical care. The scope of the study was defined as follows (Abel-Smith, 1960, p.xi):

> No attempt is made to provide a history of nursing techniques or of nursing as an activity or skill. Little is said about what it was like at different times to nurse, or to be trained as a nurse, or to receive nursing care. What the nurse was taught or who examined her are all questions which are left unanswered.

To a large extent Abel-Smith's exclusions remain valid today, and too little is known about the relationship between medical and nursing innovation and the experience of patients. Abel-Smith's volume remains an important contribution, not only for its subject matter but its style and method. It was the first to break the monopoly of 'internalist' accounts written by 'insiders' who acted as apologists for various professional causes.

Standpoints and starting points

Breaking the tradition of his predecessors, Abel-Smith does not begin his account in ancient Greece but at the turn of the nineteenth century. His definition of 'nursing' is one of paid work rather than the activity of 'caring', over which it is implied nurses have some monopolistic hold. Monica Baly's textbook on nursing and social change was originally commissioned to meet the needs of students taking the Diploma in Nursing Course of the University of London (Baly, 1973). As a 'purpose written' text it is unique, as it endeavoured for the first time to locate nursing within the wider social and economic context and enhance its relevance by discussing contemporary issues such as the nursing process.

In more recent years a modest quantity of innovative research has been published, either as edited collections such as those of Davies (1980) and Maggs (1987), or as monographs derived from post-graduate research theses.

Rosemary White's study of the neglected area of poor-law nursing was one of the first such monographs to be published in the field and helped to turn attention towards the publicly funded poor law and municipal hospitals (White, 1978). Her later work on the effect of the National Health Service (NHS) upon the nursing profession is a detailed study of the various branches and nursing organizations during the early years of the NHS (White, 1985). Although much of White's work might be located within the tradition of social administration history, more recently she has diversified into policy and organizational analyses of issues current in British and international nursing. Several of these 'case studies' have been published in a series of edited volumes concerned with various aspects of nursing policy and policies from historical and contemporary cross-cultural perspectives (White, 1985, 1986, 1987).

Much of the 'new' writing has been the product of post graduate research. Davies' (1980) edited collection was the first 'mould-breaking' collection to situate the analysis of nursing work and institutions within a revisionist tradition and to examine nursing from the point of view of the politics of class and gender. It was critical rather than congratulatory and broke new ground by including material drawn from specialisms such as mental nursing and midwifery to counteract the historiographical bias which had previously favoured general hospital nursing. Some continuity exists between

Davies' volume and Maggs' sequel (1987a) insofar as some new material continues the revisionist trend but alongside this, more familiar material and themes, including professionalization, are addressed. Further coverage of nursing specialisms is provided within a cross-cultural context, allowing useful international comparisons to be made.

Where Celia Davies has contributed towards locating nursing history on the sociological map, Christopher Maggs has helped to open up nursing history to social historians by blending social history with labour and feminist history approaches in his monograph. This examined the social composition of the nursing workforce in a cross-sectional sample of voluntary and poor-law hospitals from the late nineteenth century to the beginning of the twentieth (Maggs, 1983). Monica Baly, in her demythologizing account of the Nightingale Fund, has also helped to overturn a number of popular legends concerning the achievements of the Fund and the quality of nurse training provided under its auspices during its early years at St Thomas's hospital (Baly, 1986). Baly re-evaluates the claims to success of the Nightingale experiment and its enduring implications for the conduct of nurse education. More recently still, Anne Summers (1988), in an innovative, scholarly and eloquent study of British women as nurses from the Crimean war to World War I, has examined the politics of nursing reform within the context of women's social history, highlighting the impact of gender and class relations upon the reform endeavour. Christopher Maggs' most recent publication on the history of the Royal National Pension Fund For Nurses (Maggs, 1987b) and Monica Baly's commemorative volume on the history of the Queen's Institute (Baly, 1987) are notable, both as institutional histories and contributions to the social history of nursing.

Conclusion

History can be related to nursing in a variety of different ways and the most recent addition to the textbook market has experimented with an approach which combines the work and experience of a social historian, a sociologist and a nurse in examining nursing history (Dingwall, Rafferty and Webster, 1988). An attempt was made to integrate the application of concepts drawn from the social sciences with primary historical research and discussion of controversial contemporary issues in nursing, such as Project 2000, the impact of the Griffiths proposals upon the management of nursing work and personnel, and the rise of the nursing process and its prospects for the future.

The challenges for developing historical knowledge further in nursing are considerable and the prospects and opportunities are many and exciting. Indeed, such an undertaking invites us to consider a number of theoretical and practical issues, including the relationship between political theory and welfare and the factors and principles which determine the allocation of resources to health and health care in society at any given time. What kind of nursing care do we wish to be able to offer patients in the future? The past is inescapable but a knowledge of history will help us understand the factors which have shaped and continue to shape what one researcher of nursing has referred to as 'the art of the possible' (Menzies Lyth, 1988, pp.153–207).

References

Abel-Smith, B. (1960) *A History of the Nursing Profession*, London Heinemann

Abel-Smith, B. (1964) *The Hospitals 1800–1948*, Heinemann, London

Baly, M. (1973) *Nursing and Social Change*, Croom Helm, London

Baly, M. (1986) *Florence Nightingale and the Nursing Legacy* Croom Helm, London

Baly, M. (1987) *A History of the Queen's Institute for District Nursing: 100 Years 1887–1987*, Croom Helm, London

Bolgar, R.R. (1954) *The Classical Inheritance and its Beneficiaries*, University Press, Cambridge

Breay, M. and Bedford Fenwick, E.G. (1928–9) *History of the International Council of Nurses, 1899–1909*, International Council of Nurses Annual Reports, 1928–9, London, pp.215–275

Campbell, F. (1970) Latin and the elite tradition in education. In *Sociology: History and Education* (ed. P.W. Musgrave), Methuen, London, p. 249

Cannadine, D. (1987) British history: past, present – and future. *Past and Present*, **116**, 169–191

Christy, T. (1971) Equal rights for women. *American Journal of Nursing*, 71, 288–293

Davies C (ed.) (1980) *Rewriting Nursing History*, Croom Helm, London

Dingwall, R., Rafferty, A.M. and Webster C (1988) *An Introduction to the Social History of Nursing*, Routledge, London

Dock, L. and Stewart, I. (1920) *A Short History of Nursing*, Putnam, London

Garrison F.H. (1929) *An Introduction to the History of Medicine*, 4th edn, W.B. Saunders, Philadelphia

Kelly–Gadol, J. (1977) Did women have a Renaissance? In *Becoming Visible: Women in European History* (eds R. Bridenthal and C. Koonz), Houghton Mifflin, Boston, pp.175–202

Kropotkin, P. (1902) *Mutual Aid: a Factor in Human Evolution*, Heinemann, London

Lewis, J. (1984) *Women in England 1870–1950*, Wheatsheaf Books, London

Maggs, C.J. (1983) *The Origins of General Nursing*, Croom Helm, London

Maggs, C. J. (1987a) *Nursing History: The State of the Art*, Croom Helm, London

Maggs, C.J. (1987b) *A History of the Royal National Pension Fund*, London

Menzies Lyth, I. (1988) The welfare of children making long stays in hospital: an experiment in the art of the possible. In Menzies Lyth, I. (1988) *Containing Anxiety in Institutions*, Vol. 1, (ed. I. Menzies Lyth), Free Association Books, London

Morton, P. (1984) *The Vital Science: Biology and the Literacy Imagination 1860–1900*, Allen and Unwin, London

Nutting, A. and Dock, L. (1907–1912) *A History of Nursing*, Vols 1–4, Putnam, New York

Pavey, A.E. (1938) *The Story of the Growth of Nursing as an Art. A Vocation and a Profession*, Faber and Faber, London

Pollard, S. (1968) *The Idea of Progress: History and Society*, Watts, London

Sarnecky, M.T. (1990) Historiography: a legitimate research methodology for nursing. *Advances in Nursing Science*, **12(4)**, 1–10

Seymour, L.R. (1954) *A General History of Nursing*, Faber and Faber, London

Summers, A. (1988) *Angels and Citizens: British Women as Military Nurses 1854–1914*, Routledge, London

Thomas, K. (1983) *Man and the Natural World: Changing Attitudes in England 1500–1800*, Penguin, London

Tooley, S. (1903) *Queen Victoria*, Blousefield, London

Tooley, S. (1906) *A History of Nursing in the British Empire*, Blousefield, London

White, R. (1978) *Social Change and Development of the Nursing Profession: A Study of the Poor Law Nursing Service*, Henry Kimpton, London

White, R. (1985) *The Effects of the NHS on the Nursing Profession 1948–1960*, Oxford, King's Fund Historical Series

White, R. (1985) *Political Issues in Nursing: Past, Present and Future*, vol.1, Heinemann, London

White, R. (1986) *Political Issues in Nursing: Past, Present and Future*, vol.2, Heinemann, London

White, R. (1987) *Political Issues in Nursing: Past, Present and Future*, vol.3, Heinemann, London

Whittaker, E.W. and Olesen, V.L. (1964) The faces of Florence Nightingale: functions of the heroine legend in an occupational subculture. *Human Organisation*, **23(2)**, 123–130

Wilson, A. and Ashplant, T.G. (1988) Whig history and present-centred history. *Historical Journal*, **31(1)**, 1–16

Chapter 3

Biological perspectives

Basiro Davey

Biology is the scientific study of the structure and function of living things and of the interactions of organisms with each other in the natural world and with their environment. Biologists are supposed to be defining a set of universal laws about the nature of organisms by striving dispassionately to discover 'facts' that explain the properties of life itself. The biological tradition has been so long established that we tend to accept biological knowledge as beyond dispute. It has an aura of respectability and dependability; biologists are object-ive servants of the truth.

So pervasive is this view of biology that you might have wondered whether there is a biological debate to explore and whether this chapter might prove to be the shortest and least interesting in the book. This is in sharp contrast to psychology and sociology, the 'social' sciences that contribute most to nursing, which are relative newcomers as academic disciplines and often misrepresented as 'soft' and debatable science by comparison with the diamond-hard objectivity of 'real' science.

The expectation that biological knowledge is somehow above debate has been created by the ways in which science has traditionally been conducted and reported. Under cover of a professional smoke-screen there is abundant controversy in biology, as elsewhere in all human activities. This is not simply the predictable levels of dispute between respectful colleagues about whether we have at last got to 'the truth' of a particular question. The debate is also conducted, more or less in private, about whether biological truths are in fact qualitatively different from those of the social sciences, or are they just as liable to be subjective and biased?

The myth of objectivity

The reverence that is accorded to biological knowledge is based in part on a myth that all scientific research is an objective process, unsullied by prejudice or emotion and therefore trustworthy in some absolute sense. The scientific method of acquiring knowledge is supposed to begin with innocent and unbiased observations of real phenomena. As the results of these uninterpreted observations accumulate, patterns begin to emerge and a number of hypothetical explanations for these patterns gradually suggest themselves. The scientist who constructed these hypotheses must have no vested interest in the outcome, no preference for one hypothesis over another. He (occasionally she) simply devises more ingenious experiments to test the validity of each hypothesis and discards those that do not stand up to rigorous investigation. Even then, the surviving explanations can never be said to be proved; they cannot achieve a higher status than 'not yet disproved' for fear of the scientist becoming overly identified with a particular outcome. This is the public face of biological research and the well-spring of much of its prestige among non-scientists. It skilfully conceals the fact that all scientific knowledge is generated by human beings and is the product of social activity. It is therefore inevitable that bias, subjectivity and human error, political ideology and dogma, fashion, fancy, manipulation of results for career gain, professional jealousy, accidents and inspired hunches play a part in the conduct and reporting of biological research. From time to time the subjective nature of science is acknowledged by the very best of its exponents. Here is an extract from an essay entitled 'Is the scientific paper a fraud?' by Sir Peter Medawar (1990), one of the most influential and creative immunologists of the twentieth century and a Nobel Laureate:

> There is no such thing as unprejudiced observation. Every act of observation we make is biased. What we see or otherwise sense is a function of what we have seen or sensed in the past ... the actual formulation of a hypothesis is – let us say a guess, is inspirational in character.

The primary aim of this chapter is to convince you that biological knowledge is as debatable as any other field of human intellectual endeavour. It is relatively easy for an insider to discover compelling examples which prove that biologists have feet of clay like other men and women. This chapter concludes with some such tales. But this would be a trivial exercise without first unpacking some of the major intellectual debates about the nature of biological knowledge itself and the ways in which the research agenda has been driven by two connected ideologies. They are known as *reductionism* and *determinism*.

Reductionist versus holistic biology

Biological knowledge has been pursued since the seventeenth century from within a powerful intellectual framework known as reductionism. This is the conviction that the properties of a complex system can best be understood by separating it into smaller and smaller units of study. Biological reductionism holds that a living organism should be studied by focusing downwards through a hierarchy of organization, from the tissues and organs to the cells of which they are made, then to the molecules that are built into cells, and finally to the atoms themselves. The philosophy of reductionism ultimately states that life itself can be understood by the most detailed study of its smallest constituent parts.

This tradition has led to a very high value being placed on precision in research and on pursuing a line of investigation down through the hierarchy of biological organization at least to the molecular level. It has been a tremendously productive framework. Susan Oyama, an American psychologist and philosopher, has described it as a 'provisional single-mindedness that allows detailed investigation of a mechanism' (Oyama, 1989). But too often this provisional act of mind, which temporarily excludes the chaotic complexity of the whole, is elevated to the dominant philosophy in biological research and becomes a kind of strait-jacket which limits the kinds of question that biologists can ask and answer. Consider the following contrasting examples of the success and failure of reductionist biology. The Human Genome Project is a massive research programme involving biologists from several countries, with a budget of at least $1 billion and the task of constructing a detailed map of the 50 000–100 000 human genes and their functions within the next few decades (see

DeLisi, 1988, for a detailed discussion). And yet we cannot accurately predict or even measure the biological effects of relatively simple chemicals such as aspirin on the human body as a whole. (See Sir Peter Medawar's book *The Limits of Science*, 1986a, for an analysis of why science is good at answering some kinds of questions and inadequate for others.)

Reductionism has bred generations of biologists who think vertically rather than horizontally, who study well-defined and specialist areas in depth without paying much attention to the whole organism as a dynamic and unpredictable entity that is much more than the sum of its parts. Biological knowledge has, in accordance with the reductionist tradition, been subdivided into a number of different disciplines, each with a particular focus of interest and a rather scant acquaintance with areas of biology that fall outside it. These intellectual divisions have served the purpose of slicing an immensely complex subject into manageable chunks, but this has created a wealth of facts which conceal our ignorance about the 'big' picture.

The most fundamental division is between what might be called 'indoor' biology and 'outdoor' biology, or biological knowledge that has been generated from the study of cells and tissues in laboratories and knowledge that has been obtained by observation of animals in the natural world or in artificially created environments. At first sight, outdoor biology might appear to have very little relevance to the professional training of nurses, but a surprising number of general theories and concepts have been lifted from studies of other species and applied to the behaviour of human beings. The popularity of several books written by the biologist Desmond Morris (for example, *The Naked Ape*, 1967), testifies to the power of this tradition to influence the ways we think about ourselves as biological organisms much like our closest primate relatives.

Unless you look closely, the reductionist tradition seems weak in outdoor biology, which, by its very nature, concentrates on whole organisms, but in fact it has had a profound influence by creating an intellectual separation between the organism and the environment. If a living organism can be reduced to its component parts and these can be precisely defined, then a sharp distinction can be made between 'me' and 'not me'. From this perspective, animals, including humans, are seen as essentially different from an external world which they inhabit, even though they may act on the world and in turn are affected by external events. There are many consequences of this way of looking at the natural world, characterized most seriously by the accelerating problems of global pollution. If organisms are seen in isolation from their habitats, then it becomes possible to act on the environment without thought for the long-term effects on plant and animal life.

In recent years, a new and antireductionist philosophy has been taking shape, which might be termed 'holistic' biology because it views the organism and the environment as part of a greater whole. Consider, for a moment, the air we all breathe. The carbon dioxide that animals exhale as a waste product of their metabolism is also a raw material from which plants build complex sugars, using energy supplied by sunlight and releasing oxygen into the atmosphere as their waste product. Animals breathe the oxygen and eat the plants, using the oxygen as a fuel to break down the sugars consumed in the tissues of plants or, indirectly, in the tissues of other animals that fed on plants. Animals exhale carbon dioxide as a waste product of this process, and so the cycle goes on. So what is the air that we breathe? It is simultaneously a waste product and a food and a fuel, the molecules are constantly circulating into and out of the bodies of animals and plants, sometimes as a gas, sometimes a liquid or built into larger molecules and structured into tissues, only to be broken down again. From this perspective it is nonsense to draw a line between the organism and the atmosphere and see them as essentially different. Pollution of one is simultaneously pollution of the other.

Reductionism has had a far more apparent impact on indoor biology, which in turn has made the greatest contribution to the biological knowledge taught in schools of nursing. Laboratory biologists study the structure and functions of organisms at ever smaller hierarchical levels. Their interest encompasses the development of form in the embryo; the anatomy of the adult organism; the systems of interacting organs, macroscopic structures and tissues of which the body is made; cells of all kinds and their internal microscopic components; genes and the function of deoxyribonucleic acid (DNA); biochemical molecules and their reactions; and, ultimately, some biologists meet up with the physicists studying the intermolecular and subatomic forces that hold everything together. No individual biologist can cope with such a broad field, so there has been a long tradition of dividing laboratory research into rather separate disciplines: embryology, anatomy, physiology, cell biology, genetics, biochemistry and biophysics, to follow the same order given in the list of interest areas above.

There is a barely perceptible trend towards the gradual dissolution of these discipline boundaries and a growing recognition that a far wider range of knowledge is now needed to make further progress in research. It no longer makes such good sense to teach students about biochemistry, genetics and physiology as separate blocks of biological knowledge, as if these processes had no influence on each other in real life. The biochemical reactions that take place inside a living cell are dependent upon the genes that are active in the cell at that time and, simultaneously, the cell is affected by the physiological state of the whole animal, such that the temperature or nutritional status or water balance, the hormone levels, metabolic rate and much more, affect the biochemistry of the cell and the activation of its genes. And to hark back to the earlier discussion of the holistic philosophy, the whole organism penetrates and is penetrated by the environment of which it is a part.

But in many universities and certainly in most schools of nursing, human biology is reduced to isolated descriptions of the working parts, which are never reassembled into a human being. Biology textbooks fall into sharp disciplinary divisions, located on different shelves in the library – not surprisingly since there have been few attempts at writing holistic biology, where the whole takes precedence over the parts. (Some traditional textbooks pay more attention than most to related disciplines and a selection of the author's favourites can be found at the end of this chapter.) Moreover, the reader of traditional textbooks will obtain a biological snapshot of a standardized human being at a particular age – there are snaps of an embryo, a newborn, a child, an adolescent, a whole album full of young adults, and a few of old people – but the developmental sequence that connects them together across time is missing. We never see the whole biological trajectory, even for a standardized person, much less for an individual. Reductionism has obliterated the startling diversity hidden among the biological truths that apply to all of us. Just as our faces and fingerprints differ in subtle but unique ways, so too do our internal organs and our biochemistry, but you would never know this from a basic education in biological knowledge.

So there is an important debate in biology about the extent to which it is now time to draw back from the reductionist tradition and reconsider all its many important gifts. The modern philosophers of biology are thinking in holistic terms, but the weight of tradition is against them (see Oyama, 1989, for a comprehensive review).

Biological determinism and the 'nature–nurture' debate

Reductionism has a special application in biology because it has nourished the conviction that the state of an organism is determined by the activity of its smallest biological components. According to this ideology, every aspect of human life, from the simplest biochemical event inside a cell to the most complex outpouring of creative genius, is a direct consequence of the individual's biology and, at the ultimate level, a consequence of the individual's genes. Consider this statement by an eminent biologist (DeLisi, 1988), writing about the Human Genome Project mentioned earlier:

> This collection of chromosomes in the fertilized egg constitutes the complete set of instructions for development, determining the timing and details of the formation of the heart, the central nervous system, the immune system and every other organ and tissue required for life.

Notice that according to this deterministic view, the genetic instructions are 'the complete set' necessary for human development; in other words, 'nature' sets the agenda and controls the clock, and the world in which the person lives plays no part in shaping the outcome. This conviction has a mirror image in the most extreme forms of social or cultural determinism, which can be unearthed from time to time in certain branches of sociology and psychology and which maintain that the person is shaped entirely by his or her social relationships, entirely devoid of any inherited influence. Both positions are hard to defend, but the absolute supremacy of 'nurture' over 'nature', as argued by advocates of social determinism, is relatively easy to shoot down from everyday experience. All parents will affirm that their babies were not born as biological 'blank sheets' on which they subsequently wrote the script for how the child would develop. Children born in the same family show from the earliest age a remarkable diversity in their personality, their susceptibility to illness, their need for sleep or contact or food, their degree of alertness and so on, despite similar parenting. Against this background of apparently innate behaviour, a predictable sequence of biological development unfolds that most children follow almost regardless of 'nurture'. Even amongst malnourished infants in conditions of social deprivation, their biological development and their coordination unfolds in the normal sequence, although often severely delayed in time. Restore the child to adequate nutrition and their biological development usually catches up with children who were not deprived. The unique biological clock within each child has been ticking all the while. But it would be unthinkable to use this as evidence that the social world of children does not matter because their biology alone will determine the outcome. Or would it?

The most extreme proponents of biological determinism do indeed argue that, just as there are genes that determine the colour of a person's eyes, so too there are genes for 'aggression' or 'unselfishness' or any other trait you care to mention; you may have encountered a very popular book by biologist Richard Dawkins, *The Selfish Gene* (1976), which propounds this philosophy. Dawkins and his colleagues would not maintain that 'nurture' is irrelevant, but they argue that its influence is simply to reinforce some aspects of the genetic script that are already mapped out and to dilute others. The environment cannot create traits that are not specified in the individual's genetic programme at birth. According to this view, differences between people in terms of intelligence, athletic prowess, mathematical or artistic ability, commercial acumen and so forth, are programmed from birth by their inherited genes. It is a short hop from this biological ideology to a political one which maintains that inequality in the social order between (say) men and women, or black and white, is simply the expression of different genes and, as such, is part of an unalterable natural order. Biological knowledge of the deterministic kind has frequently been called upon as evidence for social inequality. For example, the Minister for Social Services (Patrick Jenkin, quoted in Rose, Lewontin and Kamin, 1984) speaking in 1980:

> Quite frankly, I don't think mothers have the same right to work as fathers. If the Lord had intended us to have equal rights to go to work, He wouldn't have created men and women. These are biological facts, young children do depend on their mothers.

Biological determinism is a seductive ideology because at its simplest level it appears to be true. For example, a single gene

in the human cell contains the instructions for the manufacture of an enzyme, which in turn controls the breakdown of
an amino acid called phenylalanine, a common component of
certain proteins in the diet. If the gene is faulty, then the
enzyme is faulty and large amounts of phenylalanine build up
in the body, eventually causing irreversible brain damage (the
condition is known as phenylketonuria or PKU). Babies in
Britain are routinely tested for this condition at seven days old,
before any damage is done, and put on a carefully managed
diet if PKU is detected. There is no apparent contradiction to
the deterministic view that the faulty gene causes PKU. But
does it? In the absence of phenylalanine in the diet, there
would be no way of distinguishing between people who had
the faulty gene and those who had the normal one. Indeed, the
'cure' is to change the baby's diet so that the gene becomes
irrelevant. 'Nurture' can totally counteract the effects of
'nature' in this example.

The holistic perspective on the role of genes and the
environment is that, even where the genetic composition of an
individual increases their risk of developing a certain disease,
their actual experience is influenced by an enormous range of
simultaneously and historically acting factors such as diet,
air quality, stress, reproductive history, physical activity, exposure to extremes of temperature or humidity or noise or
radiation or chemicals, contact with pathogenic organisms
and so on. A person's genes are but one factor in the equation,
not the sole determinant of the outcome. (For a superb review
of these debates, see the chapter contributed by Susan Oyama
to the *Minnesota Symposia on Child Psychology*, 1989.) One of
the most enduring claims of the biological determinists has
been for a genetic basis to mental disorders such as schizophrenia and manic depression. Indeed, a research team
believed they had located genes associated with manic depression in a closed religious sect in America, the Old Order Amish
(Egeland *et al.*, 1987), and a gene was also apparently
identified that seemed to be associated with schizophrenia in
seven British and Icelandic families with unusually high
numbers of affected members (Sherrington *et al.*, 1988). But
within two years of publication, the weight of evidence had
swung against these findings as other researchers failed to
reproduce the results. The Amish data was withdrawn as
unsound by the very group that published it originally, much
to their credit. But despite these setbacks, the conviction
remains widespread in biological circles that, given enough

time and funding, a gene that predisposes individuals to these complex conditions of the psyche will eventually be found.

None of this should be taken to mean that the genetic make-up of an individual is irrelevant to his or her experience of health and disease, or any other aspect of human life. It is simply to counsel a judicious scepticism when biology is held up as proof positive that individual lives, and hence the social structures to which they contribute, are determined by the smallest unit of biological instruction, the gene. (For a thorough critique of biological determinism and its political consequences, see Rose, Lewontin and Kamin, 1984.)

Public accounts and private practice

One area of biological knowledge of major interest to nurses is the relatively recent study of the immune system. It serves as a revealing example of some of the subjective, the political, the ethical and the financial constraints on the conduct of biological research. Immunology began in the nineteenth century with the study of resistance to infectious diseases among individuals who had recovered from a specific infection. The protective effect of vaccination had been known about since 1796, when a country doctor named Edward Jenner infected a boy with pus from a cowpox blister on the hand of a local milkmaid. Jenner subsequently exposed the boy to smallpox and demonstrated by this appallingly risky method that the boy was resistant to both diseases. It is a sobering thought that some of the most basic and important concepts in biology have been generated by experiments which, like Jenner's, would be considered totally unethical today. The debate about the ethics of acquiring biological knowledge is a topic to which we will return later.

The mechanisms underlying immunity following vaccination or recovery from infection were completely unknown until well into the nineteenth century and only dimly understood until the 1950s and 1960s. Soon after World War II, research into skin grafting the victims of wartime burns revealed that the mechanisms that rejected foreign skin grafts were the same as those that destroyed foreign organisms infecting the body. Since that time, much progress in understanding these mechanisms has been made. It has taken the pooled knowledge of physiology, genetics and biochemistry in particular to generate a description of the cells, molecules and processes that maintain our immune defences and enabled their manipulation in the service of human health. This understanding has made blood transfusions, the grafting of skin and even the transplanting of major organs from person to person a commonplace event in Western medicine. Vaccines have been developed which give protection against some of the world's most feared diseases: smallpox, for example, was declared officially eradicated from the world in 1980.

Biological histories such as this one tend to be reported in just these heroic terms, which reinforce the prestige and apparent invulnerability of biological knowledge. The achievements of famous men (rarely women) are documented. Progress seems to have marched onward inexorably towards success, the objectivity of the research method guarded by dispassionate scientists who sought the truth in the service of humanity. Yet this triumphal account leaves out a great deal of guesswork, failure, frustration and even a few lies. The omissions illustrate very clearly the profound difference between the private practice of all biological research and the public dissemination of the knowledge that it generates. Some of what we now know (or believe we know) about the immune system was stumbled over by accident: experiments 'went wrong' and were subsequently found to have produced puzzling results which led to further and fruitful investigation; researchers in other fields dabbled a bit outside their usual area of interest on a slack day and spotted the clue that others had sought diligently for years. Here is Sir Peter Medawar again, writing in his autobiography (Medawar, 1986b) about a particular research project:

> The research that I now began followed up a chance discovery . . . if mice were fed for a week or two upon a diet of commercial 'mouse-cake' heated to above 120°C by steam under pressure, they became highly reactive immunologically and threw off skin grafts transplanted from mice of different strains much more vigorously than mice reared upon the conventional diet. From this observation I was led by what I can now clearly see to have been a series of unsound inferences to form the opinion that certain derivatives of vitamin A have the power to boost the immunological response. It is not the most important research that we are engaged upon but I recount it in some detail because it is so characteristic of the way a research project starts and takes shape.

In sharp contrast to this haphazard process, biological research is written and published as though an unbroken sequence of logical deduction from objective observations had taken place. In his essay on the traditional form of the scientific research paper, Medawar attacked the 'fraud' of reporting the observations and results as though the author had no passion or prejudice in the outcome. In reality, the researcher began with an inspired hunch which shaped the choice of experiments and drove the investigation forward from its concealed location in the author's mind. Medawar (1990) advocated a new form of scientific writing in which the scientist starts by divulging his or her hypotheses and goes on to state how these ideas were tested.

> Scientists should not be ashamed to admit, as many of them apparently are ashamed to admit, that hypotheses appear in their minds along uncharted byways of thought.

Scientists are also rather hesitant to admit that the great bulk of research effort has never been published. Vast amounts of time and energy and money have been poured into lines of enquiry that produced absolutely nothing of worth, or so it seemed at the time. Later generations may go back over the same ground and find it littered with unnoticed clues. And behind the scenes, careers were being made or broken, projects were pursued or abandoned for personal rather than scientific reasons, or sometimes the money simply dried up. Productive research has often been abandoned unfinished because those who held the purse-strings diverted the funding to other projects. In 1990, the Medical Research Council closed down a successful UK laboratory which was investigating the survival of tissues at very low temperatures, an area considered to be essential for creating a 'bank' of organ transplants. One of the financial beneficiaries was the expanding acquired immune deficiency syndrome (AIDS) research programme. So progress in biological knowledge can be profoundly affected by decisions taken at the highest levels of the few key organizations with power over the flow of money: one area of research is dried up while a more fashionable area is lubricated.

And what of the lies? In a notorious case in the 1970s, an eminent American immunologist claimed to have developed a technique for radically improving the survival of foreign skin grafts in mice, by culturing the graft in a tank of nutrient medium for a number of days before grafting it on to its new host. He displayed white mice with healthy patches of black skin, apparently as a result of this manipulation, and a breakthrough in transplant technology was hailed. But within weeks his colleagues became suspicious and it was subsequently confirmed that the transplanted skin was in fact from white mice that were genetic 'twins' to the recipient mouse, hence the success of the graft. The black coloration was supplied by injections of ink. Disgrace and retraction of the published research followed, but this unsavoury story must be viewed as the tip of a (hopefully) small iceberg of fake biological knowledge that has not yet been uncovered.

It also illustrates another aspect of the search for new biological knowledge: the pressure on individual biologists to publish a steady stream of interesting results or lose his or her place in the queue for funding. In the USA, the majority of research staff are employed on fixed-term contracts, even at the most senior level, so scientists have about three years to produce sparkling work or find themselves out of a job. It is no wonder then that research activity is frantic, people start early and work late, and the competition between laboratories with similar goals can resemble limited warfare. In such an atmosphere, the sharing of results is an anathema until every last detail is ready for publication. Everyone has stories to tell in private about the assistant who turned out to be a spy from a rival laboratory, or the seminar given to an in-house audience at which three strangers were detected at the back writing it all down at furious speed.

Usually the knowledge of such rivalry is kept 'in the family', but occasionally it spills out and makes a public splash. A famous recent example is the dispute between two rival biologists who both claimed to be the first to isolate the human immunodeficiency virus (HIV), the causative agent of AIDS. Luc Montagnier in France and Robert Gallo in the USA published their results in 1984, and a vigorous battle ensued about who had prior claim to this particularly lucrative piece of biological knowledge. The prizes were immense: the prestige of winning an important academic race; the additional research funding that would certainly follow; and the patent rights to a blood testing kit that each laboratory had developed for commercial use. The patent was originally awarded to Gallo, but Montagnier proved that he had submitted a patent claim to the US Patent and Trademark Office seven months earlier than Gallo. Moreover, Gallo had been sent a sample of the French virus isolated by Montagnier a few months before both laboratories published their results. The French were suspicious, but Gallo claimed that he had not used Montagnier's sample in developing the blood test kit and that he had isolated the virus himself from American samples.

In 1988, lawyers representing the two sides reached a settlement that effectively rewrote the scientific history of the case. Henceforth, Montagnier and Gallo are deemed to have isolated the virus simultaneously and to have submitted a joint patent application for the blood testing kit. Eighty per cent of the royalties from the sale of these kits is now paid into a foundation that supports AIDS research, managed by six trustees drawn equally from the French and American research institutes concerned in the original dispute. It is reassuring that a quarter of the income is earmarked for AIDS research in 'the less developed countries of the world', since the annual royalties from HIV test kits are well in excess of $5 million.

The purpose of recounting such a tale is not simply to amuse the reader but to call into question the validity of the widespread misconception that all science is a dispassionate business in which honourable men and women seek after truth and publish it fearlessly and without hope of gain. Biological knowledge may once have been like that, but no longer. Human health and the prevention or alleviation of disease are very big business indeed and nowhere is the potential for profit greater than in the field of genetic engineering. Financial reward is bound up with one of the most heated biological debates: the ethical constraints on acquiring biological knowledge.

Biological knowledge and the ethical debate

Genetic engineering goes way beyond the possible limits of animal or plant breeding, which selects desirable characteristics and increases their expression in successive generations. It is now common practice for biological research laboratories to take out patents on living cells that have been tampered with to alter their genes and hence direct the biochemical output of the cell. Bacteria, in particular, have proved to be fruitful hosts for genes snipped from the chromosomes of other species and spliced into the bacterial deoxyribonucleic acid (DNA). Thus, for example, the gene that directs human cells to manufacture insulin has been introduced into bacteria, which are grown in huge vats that become insulin 'factories'. Diabetics have benefited significantly from this inexhaustible source, which has replaced the variable quality and sometimes serious side-effects of former insulin supplies extracted from pigs and other domestic species. These bacteria are protected by patent, just as some livestock which have been 'improved' by the introduction of genes from other species are protected.

There is something inherently disturbing to many people about taking out a patent on a form of life. Although the biological community is vigorously engaged in the moral debate and has set international safeguards against unscrupulous or dangerous exploitation of this new knowledge, there is undoubtedly concern about possible abuses of genetic engineering. Experiments which flout the guidelines have been detected, including some conducted by Western researchers in Third World countries out of reach of the supervision required by the safety code.

Stranger still is the case of Helen Lane, a young American woman who died of cancer more than twenty years ago. Some of her cancer cells were kept in tissue culture, where they divided repeatedly if supplied with nutrients. The cells were allowed to multiply and became a valuable source of cancer cells for research purposes. These HeLa cells (named after the patient) have been donated to cancer research laboratories around the world, where they are used in a variety of experiments. They are a commercially as well as a biologically useful research tool and have become the subject of legal battles. Relatives of the dead woman have claimed a stake in the profits arising from the use of these cells; the research laboratories have counter-claimed that the HeLa cells existing today are such distant descendants from the originals taken from Helen Lane that they are no longer 'hers' in any personal sense.

These examples raise profoundly controversial questions about the ethics of altering living cells in order to reap certain benefits, some of which are undoubtedly the alleviation of suffering or hunger, but there is also the huge profit to be made from some types of biological experiment. Similar ethical concerns have also been expressed about biological research into *in vitro* fertilization (IVF), in which ova are removed from a woman's body, fertilized in cell cultures and allowed to develop for several days before reintroducing the tiny embryo into her uterus. This technique has had a limited but much publicized success in overcoming certain kinds of infertility, and has other applications, for example in enabling the selection of a genetically normal embryo for implantation in cases of high probability of genetic disease. IVF generates 'surplus' embryos because the drugs given to induce ovulation produce multiple ova and it is potentially dangerous to return all the resultant embryos to the mother in case multiple pregnancies occur. Should these extra embryos be destroyed at once, or can they be used in strictly regulated research aimed at increasing biological knowledge of embryonic development, which in turn may improve the success rate of IVF? Now that the UK Parliament has agreed to certain limited research uses of human embryos up to fourteen days of development, this particular ethical debate is one that directly confronts nurses who work in infertility clinics.

Finally, there are ethical and functional debates about the uses of animals in biological research. Can the suffering of a limited number of (say) mice or monkeys be justified in order to maximize the chances of improving the health of human beings? To what extent are the results of biological research carried out on one species capable of extrapolation to another? What are the limitations of research on cell or tissue cultures, as opposed to research on whole animals?

The translation of biological knowledge into nursing practice

It is appropriate to conclude this hymn to strategic scepticism by turning to the daily practice of a nurse's work. Biology is one of the cornerstones of nursing practice (as it is in medicine, which is equally trusting of biological 'truths'). Basic training includes a wide range of biological facts and figures, which are translated into some aspect of practice. For example, nurses learn the physiological mechanisms that enable people to regulate their body temperature at close to 37 °C, or their blood pressure at around 120/80 mmHg, or to exclude sugar from their urine. Thereafter, the rationale for taking a patient's temperature, or blood pressure, or sugar-testing their urine is understood in terms of the patient's ability to maintain these biological 'norms'. Deviations from the accepted values are considered to be possible signs of underlying pathology. All this sounds pretty straightforward until you reflect on the fact that even the most senior nurses do not usually read biological research journals, so advances in biological knowledge are slow to enter the nursing curriculum. Furthermore, the biologists who study human physiology do not usually do so in health care settings.

The biological definition of 'normal' blood pressure, say, is based on measurements taken from apparently healthy volunteers under ideal resting and exercise conditions. We do not know what the 'normal' range of blood pressure might be for a distressed 8-year-old who has just seen her mother leave the children's ward at the end of visiting time; yet if the hour for a routine check has struck, then the measurement will be made regardless of biological knowledge about its meaning. Nurses cannot turn to a biological literature on the effects of a long bus ride and a noisy waiting room on blood pressure in the elderly patient, even though the consequences may be profound. Here is an extract from an article in the *British Medical Journal* by a leading specialist in the epidemiology of coronary heart disease (Rose, 1981):

> A general practitioner, say, makes a routine measurement of a man's blood pressure and finds it raised. Thereafter both the man and the doctor will say that he 'suffers' from high blood pressure. He walks in a healthy man but he walks out a patient, and his new-found status is confirmed by the giving and receiving of tablets. An inappropriate label has been accepted because both public and profession feel that if the man were not a patient the doctor would have no business treating him.

A great deal of routine nursing (and medical) practice is founded on the assumption that biological knowledge about population norms for certain physiological parameters is above dispute and can therefore be transferred to every patient in every situation. The 4-hourly TPR and BP take up a huge amount of nursing time for dubious benefit and at some inconvenience to the patient in many cases (see Burroughs and Hoffbrand, 1990, for a review), but the rationale for such work is an uncritical acceptance of biological data. The aim of this chapter has been to demystify biological knowledge by unpacking some of the most significant debates and taking you behind the scenes to reveal something of how biological research is conducted in private. Biology makes an extremely important contribution to knowledge for nursing, but it merits no more and no less reverence than any other product of our intellectual activity.

References

Burroughs, J. and Hoffbrand, B.l. (1990). A critical look at nursing observations. *Postgraduate Medical Journal*, **66**, 370–372

Dawkins, R. (1976) *The Selfish Gene*, Oxford University Press, New York

DeLisi, C. (1988) The human genome project. *American Scientist*, **76**, 488–493

Egeland, J.A., Gerhard, D.S., Pauls, D.L. *et al.* (1987) Bipolar affective disorders linked to DNA markers on chromosome 11. *Nature*, **325**, 783–787

Medawar, P. (1986a) *The Limits of Science*, University Press, Oxford

Medawar, P. (1986b) *Memoir of a Thinking Radish: An Autobiography*, University Press, Oxford, pp. 228–233

Medawar, P. (1990) Is the scientific paper a fraud? In *The Threat and the Glory* (ed. D. Pyke), University Press, Oxford

Morris, D. (1967) *The Naked Ape*, Jonathan Cape, London

Oyama, S. (1989). Ontogeny and the central dogma: do we need the concept of genetic programming in order to have an evolutionary perspective? In *Systems and Development* (eds M.R. Gunnar and E. Thelen), *The Minnesota Symposia on Child Psychology*, **22**, 1–34, Lawrence Erlbaum, Hillsdale NJ

Rose, G. (1981) Strategy of prevention: lessons from cardiovascular disease. *British Medical Journal*, **282**, 1847–1851

Rose, S., Lewontin, R.C. and Kamin, L.J. (1984) *Not in Our Genes*, Pelican, London

Sherrington, R., Brynjolfsson, J., Petursson H. *et al.* (1988) Localisation of a susceptibility locus for schizophrenia on chromosome 5. *Nature*, **336**, 164–167

Further Reading

Geleherter, T.D. and Collins F.S. (1990) *Principles of Medical Genetics*, Williams and Wilkins, Baltimore

Guyton, A.C. (1981) *Textbook of Medical Physiology*, 6th edn, W.B. Saunders Philadelphia

Macleod, A. and Sikora, K. (eds) (1984) *Molecular Biology and Human Disease*, Blackwell Scientific, Oxford

Roitt, I., Brostoff, J. and Male, D. (1990) *Immunology*, 2nd edn, Churchill Livingstone, London

Rose, S.P.R. (1991) *The Chemistry of Life*, Penguin, London

Chapter 4
Sociological perspectives

Kate Robinson

Describing his teaching of sociology to medical students, Armstrong (1982) comments that change, consolidation or confusion in the beliefs of the students are all acceptable learning outcomes. It could be said that Armstrong's students are getting good value: any student of sociology who does not experience confusion is probably being short-changed! Nursing students, however, often find this uncomfortable and criticize sociology and the other social sciences for being overly complex and lacking certainty (see, for example, Dingwall, 1977). So what is the relationship between sociology and nursing?

Sociology is the scientific study of society and it is therefore not surprising to find that there is a self-conscious relationship between nursing and sociology; nurses are informed by sociological work and 'borrow' or 'mine' sociological ideas and concepts to develop as part of nursing knowledge. The exact nature of this relationship has been explored in a number of books and articles which will be reviewed later, but it is a central theme of this book that such mining should include an understanding of the intellectual and historical context of the discipline being mined. And, as a generalization, it is fair to say that nurses have not sufficiently concerned themselves with the complexity of sociological thought before adopting and using such concepts as role, class and bureaucracy.

Sociologists are concerned with how individuals interact with each other in society, and particularly with the idea that people both have free will to act how they please and yet are constrained by social structures. We understand fairly clearly, if crudely, how the law of gravity constrains us, but the complex ways in which social structures constrain what we do are not yet understood. Sociologists are interested in social organization: the reasons why society works as it does and the consequences of it being organized in particular ways. Interest in social organization was generated by the processes of industrialization and the ways in which our society has been shaped by conflicts of class; now, of course, we need to consider the consequences of living in a post industrial society. But such matters are, of course, also within the domain of history, economics and psychology. Indeed they are the concern of everyone in a common-sense way, so what is special about sociology? How does sociological knowledge of society differ from the sort of knowledge that everybody needs in order to function competently as a member of society.

In a very well-known book, *Invitation to Sociology*, Peter Berger (1966, pp.27–28) offered the following definition:

> The sociologist, then, is someone concerned with understanding society in a disciplined way. The nature of this discipline is scientific. This means that what the sociologist finds and says about the social phenomenon he studies occurs within a rather strictly defined frame of reference. One of the main characteristics of this scientific frame of reference is that operations are bound by certain rules of evidence.

Sociological work can therefore be defined by both the specific focus of interest *and* by the methods which are used to reach conclusions about how people act together; about what evidence is considered legitimate and how conclusions are drawn. This might seem to imply that sociology is essentially an empirical discipline based on extensive practical research, but this is not the whole story. In order to generate research, sociologists need to consider possible models of society, to consider how things might be, in order to contrast that with what they find. Sociology is therefore about theory and empirical study (Murcott, 1989, p.84):

> What, of course, should distinguish sociology is that, *at one and the same time* it is the principled, thought-out (theorized) systematic and deliberate (empirical) study of the social. Good sociology keeps theory, method and the substantive simultaneously in view. Poor sociological work is often inferior precisely because it concentrates over-long on one or another.

However, these two aspects, the theoretical and the empirical, have in practice been pulled apart. Mills (1959) pointed out that there was a division between those pursuing theoretical questions, such as Parsons, and those involved in atheoretical research, such as Lazersfeld. While Payne *et al.* (1981) have suggested that this division was not so extreme in British sociology as in American, much of sociological writing can be viewed as a history of relatively untested ideas about the nature of society. This emphasis on theoretical issues rather than substantive research is reinforced in the ways in which sociology is taught: many courses focus strongly on relating the history of the discipline (see the critique ofered by Payne *et al.*, 1981; Silverman, 1981); consequently many textbooks, which are, of course, written for sociology students, spend time on summaries of the ideas of the 'founding fathers', that is Comte, Marx, Durkheim and Weber, and later commentators such as Parsons. It is very difficult indeed to relate many of these ideas about society to particular situations or to suggest ways in which they can be tested by empirical research as they are expressed at a high level of generality.

Sociological empirical research has therefore tended to proceed independently in trying to solve the smaller-scale problems which present themselves and which researchers are funded to address. So there is a division in sociology between, as Payne *et al.* (1981) put it, those who *do* sociology and those who *think about* sociology. (Until recently a similar distinction predominated within nursing.) However, doing sociology is itself far from unproblematic as there is little general agreement amongst sociologists about exactly how it should be done, or perhaps more precisely how we might know things. These disagreements relate to the theoretical discussions but not in a direct fashion; the theoretical sociological debates inform rather than direct the epistemological ones.

Sociology began by emulating the research process and logic of the natural sciences, an approach known as positivism. However, it became apparent that such methods cannot adequately deal with the fact that sociologists both study and *are* people. As Payne *et al.* (1981, p.46) state:

Put at its simplest, sociologists have become exercised by the problem that, as social beings themselves, they import their previous experiences, socialization, attitudes and beliefs into the social setting that they study.

The reformists have a number of responses to the perceived difficulties of positivism, some asserting that the standards of verification relevant to the natural sciences are not relevant to the social sciences, others proposing that such standards do not in any case reflect the reality of any sort of scientific activity. Unfortunately, this important debate has tended to become polarized into two opposing positions: positivism, which links sociological work strongly to the methods and views of the natural sciences, and interpretive sociology, which is concerned to understand situations from the perspective of the participants. These two perspectives are sometimes referred to as 'the view from above' (positivism) and 'the view from within' (interpretive sociology).

The theoretical perspectives which will inform the work of the researchers will be derived from sociological theorists. They are commonly grouped for the purposes of textbooks, into at least four perspectives. These are:

- Structural functionalism
- Conflict functionalism (Marxism)
- Symbolic interactionism
- Ethnomethodology.

For practical purposes the boundaries are much less clear-cut and researchers may well draw on more than one tradition. But as a generalization, sociologists working within each of these perspectives will almost certainly favour different methods of collecting and analysing research data, but the differences between them are not simply a matter of methods. In essence, they disagree about the way the social world is, about how people work and act in it. Functionalists, for example, see that people can be acted upon by social forces outside of their control. They have analysed the way in which, for example, people's class will affect many aspects of their lives. Symbolic interactionists and ethnomethodologists, in contrast, have focused on the individual as a prime mover in the social world. Interactions are often a major focus of their inquiry.

In part, the differences are a product of the intellectual history of Europe and the United States. Sociology does not exist in isolation from other intellectual work, and ideas from outside have impinged on sociologists and generated new sociological thinking. Ethnomethodology, for example, which is a recent perspective generated by Garfinkel (1967), can be linked to work in linguistics and philosophy, notably the later writings of Wittgenstein, as well as to the work of Parsons.

While researchers will not necessarily pledge overt allegiance to any perspective, Cuff and Payne (1979) argue that it will be demonstrated in any particular piece of work by the:

- Assumptions which are being made
- Type of questions being asked
- Concepts being used to ask the question
- Methods being used to find out about the world
- Types of answers or solutions or explanations which are accepted as valid answers to the questions being asked.

Specialist areas

The third part of the trilogy of sociology is the substantive area; Denzin, for example, refers to the three related activities of theory, research and substantive interest (Denzin, 1977). Specialist interests tend to change over time as areas come into and out of academic fashion. Payne *et al.* (1981) identify those areas predominant at some time in British sociology during the 1960s and 1970s as education, gender, law, sociolinguistics and work. Notable omissions they define as the family, population, religious affiliation and political power. Which substantive areas are included and which ones neglected is not of course simply a product of the various interests of sociologists, although this may be a factor. It reflects the complexity of the funding and organizational context of sociology. Sociology is an enterprise which needs to be funded, either as part of a teacher's job, in which case the research will have to fit around teaching commitments, or as a separate activity done within governmental or private institutions and for a number of purposes. And of course the source of funding is reflected in the areas of research. It is not just coincidence that, as Payne *et al.* assert, 'Electors have been studied rather than cabinets, just as trade unions have been studied rather than boards of directors.'

These specialist areas will be reflected in textbooks on sociology – such books can, after all, only report on work which has been done – although textbooks also reflect the presumed interest of the targeted readers. Goldthorpe (1985), for example, in an introduction to sociology intended for a mainly African readership, has chapters on kinship, marriage and the family; technology, economy and society; social class; aggression, conflict and social control; magic, religion and society. While these topics also appear in a textbook intended for use in the college system of the USA (Leslie, Larson and Gorman, 1980), there is more emphasis on sex roles, deviance, mass communication, bureaucracy and minorities, specifically 'Blacks in the United States'.

Neutrality or commitment

Sociology is a science of people: it analyses and defines people's condition. How far then do its practitioners have a commitment to change any of the situations which they document? In the nineteenth century, Marx, stated that: 'Philosophers have variously interpreted the world. The point, however, is to change it.' But how far is this a consistent theme of contemporary sociologists? Becker, discussed this issue in a famous article: 'Whose side are we on?' and argued that the researcher must inevitably adopt a particular perspective from which to view a situation (Becker, 1970, p.131):

> A student of medical sociology may decide that he will take neither the perspective of the patient nor the perspective of the physician, but he will necessarily take a perspective that impinges on the many questions which arise between physicians and patients; no matter what perspective he takes, his work will either take into account the attitude of subordinates or it will not.

The problem of commitment has been highlighted from another quarter. Delamont, in her work *The Sociology of Women: An Introduction* (Delamont, 1980), argued that sociology has largely ignored issues of sex and gender; that these, unlike issues of class, insofar as they had been considered at all, had been seen as natural, as within the biological domain, and therefore not part of the legitimate focus of sociology. In her view (Delamont, 1980, pp.6–7):

> Almost all of the sociologists of the last 150 years have built theories about society as a whole, and about women, around unexamined myths and beliefs concerning the two sexes common in their own time and culture, rather than subjecting these beliefs to critical scrutiny or engaging in thorough research ... Sociology has been unscholarly and sexist.

Following previous work, Delamont argues that:

- Important areas of social enquiry have been overlooked.

- There has been emphasis on the public, visible domain, to the exclusion of the less obvious private domain.
- The issue of sex and gender has not been taken seriously in research design, for example, that male sociologists may not have access to certain kinds of information.
- Sex is not sufficiently seen as a factor which can explain the phenomena under investigation.
- Sociology may assume a 'single society' in which a generalization can be taken to apply to all.

Importantly, she allies herself (Delamont, 1980, p.11) to the idea that:

> Sociology frequently explains the status quo (and therefore helps provide rationalizations for existing power distributions), yet social science should explore needed social transformations and encourage a more just, humane society.

Sociology of health and illness

The branch of sociology which is now known as the sociology of health and illness is just one of the specialist areas of sociology which both contribute to and draw their inspiration from the major issues of sociological theory and research practice. As a specialist area of interest it has a number of roots and it could be said that it remains a rather uneasy alliance of interests. The roots are embedded in sociology, social policy and social anthropology. First, there is the work of sociologists who studied health care as a byproduct of other interests. Dingwall's study of health visitor training (Dingwall, 1977), for example, which includes some description and analysis of health visitor knowledge and practice, grew out of an interest in the processes of education rather than of health care.

Second, the demands of teaching sociology within the medical syllabus produced interest in what work was and was not relevant, and stirred consciousness of it as a subject. Textbooks were required to cover the curriculum, and the production of such books led to the creation of a self-conscious body of knowledge. Third, interest in health care has been a major part of the social policy critiques which are concerned with issues of social welfare. Since Beveridge identified health as one of the five pillars of a welfare state, any evaluation of inequality of provision will incorporate a review of health care. Fourth, a concern with the apparent rising costs and diminishing returns of health care has encouraged both interest and funding in the areas particularly of health care organizations and people's illness behaviour. In the USA, in particular, there is considerable concern about the viability of the health care system: Conrad and Kern, for example, writing in 1981 talk about the 'crisis' in USA health care.

The sociology of health and illness is now a self-conscious discipline or specialty, as measured by a number of criteria. Within the UK, for example, there are undergraduate and postgraduate courses in the sociology of health and illness; there is a British Sociological Association (BSA) interest group which holds a conference each year and distributes the newsletter *Medical Sociology News*. There is also a major UK journal *Sociology of Health and Illness*. The major debates within sociology as a whole, such as issues of what substantive areas to address, what methods to choose to address them, and in whose interests sociological work should be done, have also been actively pursued within the context of the sociology of health and illness.

However, one of the major internal debates has centred around the primary focus of the specialty, and consequently what its title should be. Two decades ago the use of the title '*Medical Sociology*' was still common and reflected a major focus both on the activities of doctors in the health care system and the needs of doctors in training for input from sociologists. It is clear from reading the introductions to medical sociology textbooks that a claim was being made that medicine was an applied discipline which should be at least as dependent on the social sciences as on the natural sciences (see, for example, Freeman, Levine and Reeder, 1972). However, the move to the broader conceptualization of the area as the sociology of health and illness was perhaps less radical than it appeared. Conrad and Kern (1981), for example, argue towards a reorientation on the grounds that sociology *in* medicine had been neglected in favour of sociology *of* medicine. This distinction was first made by Strauss in 1957: sociology in medicine was defined as being concerned with the application of sociology to the ecology and aetiology of disease and variations in attitude and behaviour regarding health and illness, and the sociology of medicine as concerned with issues such as the recruitment and training of physicians and medical organizations (Kendall and Reader, 1972). The former suggests a discipline which is concerned essentially with medical questions, the latter with sociological ones. While the concerns of the sociology of medicine can be construed as attempts to redefine the area of illness as social, they would not necessarily include a substantial critique of the role of health care organizations and workers and an examination of lay health workers – issues which have been raised in a recent major textbook in the field which attempts to move the ground once more by using the title *A Sociology of Health and Healing* (Stacey, 1988). Stacey (1988, p.1) is concerned with:

> the arrangements that are and have been made at different times and places for restoring and maintaining health and for ameliorating suffering, paying particular attention to biomedicine in advanced industrial societies and most specifically in Britain.

She is particularly interested in emphasizing the contribution all members of a society make to health production and maintenance; that the patient is a health worker, and that the characteristics of 'human service' or 'people work' distinguish it from other social activities. She uses the arena of health care to generate theories about the distinctions in our society, notably the gender order, age distinctions and the public/private domain.

This more radical approach to the subject moves away from the competition for expertise in health care into a broader conceptualization of what health care is. Within such a conceptualization formal health care services are shifted away from the centre of the health and illness stage. Interestingly, neither this formulation, nor the previous more medically oriented one, pays much attention to nurses and nursing. However, there is the potential within Stacey's broader perspective to explore issues of the relationship between lay and 'professional' nursing and nurses. Such questions may be increasingly important as changes in the health service orient the responsibility for care increasingly towards friends and relatives in the community.

Sociology and nursing

While the advent of the redefinition and reorganization of nursing undertaken by the statutory bodies in the 1980s, and known as Project 2000, may have brought sociology firmly within the realms of nursing education, the idea that sociological knowledge is important in nursing is not a new one. In the late 1970s a number of authors set out to explore the relationship between nursing and sociology (Chapman, 1976; Smith, 1976; Cox, 1979). Cox, in her paper entitled *Who cares? Nursing and sociology: the development of a symbiotic relationship*, chooses four areas of sociological work which have been particularly useful to nursing. These are:

- Changing patterns of disease, dependency and death
- Social and cultural variations in perceptions of, and responses to, disease
- Organizational analyses
- Sociological studies of interpersonal relationships.

The contribution of nursing to this 'symbiotic relationship' is defined as the provision of interesting data for sociological analyses.

More recently, Theodore (1989, p.74) has argued that:

> The aims of any sociological dimension should not be to burden our students with esoteric knowledge or to achieve academic respectability for the nursing programme. The principal aims should be:

- To explore sociological issues and the implications for nursing practice.
- To enable the students to be more sensitive to clients' problems and needs.
- To increase personal awareness of social factors.
- To help students to realize that social factors influence patient and nurse equally.

Within such perspectives, the role of sociology in general terms has been largely limited to explaining the world to the nurse so that, so the logic runs, she can offer a better service. The world of the nurse, however, is not part of the vision; complex analysis of nursing as work has not either been required of sociologists or been noticeably forthcoming.

Health care workers will gain knowledge of sociology from two sources. First, there is the literature of sociology itself: texts written primarily for sociologists to add to the corpus of sociological knowledge. Second, there are the introductory textbooks written specifically for that purpose. Melia (19xx), in a review of introductory texts for health care workers, suggests that there are major problems with this approach. It represents a compromise between the interests of the discipline, which requires that the ideas are presented with some complexity and with explanation of the processes by which analysis was developed, and the needs of the student who will have few skills, and probably little time, with which to tackle the subject. There is a danger that any text produced under such conditions will be little more than a 'shopping list' of topics, an approach which reduces the credibility of the subject. As Melia (1986, p.88) argues:

> Ultimately this approach robs sociology's insights of any theoretical basis and does the discipline a gross disservice. The net result is a collection of sociological and anthropological facts which, whilst they may be of some practical use, will not appear to the medical or nursing student to be particularly different from any number of other facts which they learn and draw upon – normal values of physiological measurements, drug dosages, etc.

Sociologists themselves are not unaware of this problem. Mechanic, writing in 1968, includes this note in the Introduction (pp.10–11):

> The purpose of a general book such as this one is to define an area of study, and to give readers some perspective on the issues that concern investigators, the knowledge and understanding they have gleaned, and some of the problems that remain to be effectively attacked. Because such books are not specific to any single issue, but rather cover a large range of issues, they tend to simplify complex and difficult matters, and to treat issues as resolved and facts as known which in reality are continuously being debated among researchers working in the specific fields concerned. Such general treatments not infrequently confuse hypothesis with fact, and impressions with confirmation. If a general book is written in the same fashion as a critical monograph, it is likely to fail in its task of presenting a perspective and a 'feel of the field' for the general student, but if a general book is not sensitive to controversies concerning facts in its field, it may easily perpetuate incorrect ideas and even 'educated nonsense' under the guise of learning. Thus such a book, if it is to meet its responsibilities to its field, cannot be free of uncertainties, disagreements, and technical issues which have a direct bearing on the facts.

This general critique should form a very useful reference for the student choosing from the increasing range of relevant textbooks in library or bookshop.

Conclusion

Throughout this chapter I have been focusing on the internal disputes – in Rex's terms the Wars of Religion of sociology – which, reflected in sociology texts of various kinds, limit the accessibility of sociological thinking to 'outsiders' such as nurses. In the immediately preceding section, it was suggested that attempts to summarize or contain the richness of socio-logical thinking are inevitably futile. In this final section it is therefore important to change the focus and ask the question: 'Why, then, should nursing maintain and develop a relation-ship with sociology?' This question has not been well an-swered by nurses themselves, but Payne *et al.* (1981, p.280) offer both a broad view of the value of sociological research, and presumably the consequent dissemination of knowledge for any occupation, and a 'worked example' in the field of child care. The generalization runs as follows:

> This justification has to rest in the sociological imagination, the ability to transcend the boundaries of one particular interest . . . [occupational groups] are limited, however, in their ability to question their own terms of reference.

Their discussion of child care, and particularly child abuse, identifies four specific ways in which a sociologist could contribute to the interests of practitioners. First, the question 'Is this a real problem?' could be asked. Problems, as we all know, have fashions and may be creatures of media 'hype' or artefacts of changed statistics; it is important to consider these issues before investing resources in the search for solutions. Second, the sociologist can supply realistic figures on the incidence of the problem which can be used as a basis for accurate planning. Third, he or she can discover what patterns of family organization relate to the problem of child abuse. Fourth, and possibly the most important to practitioners, he or she can investigate how any planned intervention might work in practice. We are increasingly familiar with examples of how intervention in nature (building a dam, constructing a road, introducing a new species) can have catastrophic con-sequences which were not foreseen. Social interventions can be equally catastrophic – even if they simply do not work they will have consumed resources which could have been invested elsewhere – and the sociologists can assist in analysing the potential effects of the intervention. Such an analysis could be applied in very many situations in nursing, which is an occupation increasingly prone to adopting unresearched organizational and therapeutic changes on a wide scale.

However, in conclusion it is worth re-emphasizing one of the realities of sociology which will not go away, however much nurses and other occupational groups might wish it, and that is that it will not become neater and tidier. As Hawthorne (1876, p.259), cited in Payne *et al.* (1981), states:

> Sociology will remain as it is and always has been [a] very disorderly and wholly provisional enterprise ... [because] it rests on philosophical anthropology, upon a view of what men (sic) are and may be that is essentially contestable.

This should be perceived, however, as a strength of the discipline, not a weakness.

Acknowledgements

I would like to thank Robert Dingwall, Martin O'Brien and Pam Watson for commenting on an earlier draft of this chapter.

References and further reading

Armstrong, D. (1982) The way we teach medical sociology. In *Handbook for Sociology Teachers* (eds R. Gomm and P. McNeil), Heinemann, London, pp.285–289

Becker, H.S. (1970) *Sociological Work*, Aldine, Chicago

Berger P. (1966) *Invitation to Sociology*, Penguin, London

Chapman, C.M. (1976) The use of sociological theories and models in nursing. *Journal of Advanced Nursing*, 1,111–127

Chapman, C.M. (1977) *Sociology for Nurses*, Baillière Tindall, London

Conrad, P. and Kern, R. (eds) (1981) *The Sociology of Health and Illness: Critical Perspectives*, St Martin's Press, New York

Cox, C. A. (1979) Who cares? Nursing and sociology: the development of a symbiotic relationship. *Journal of Advanced Nursing*, 4, 237–252

Cox, C. (1984) *Sociology: An Introduction for Nurses, Midwives and Health Visitors*, Butterworths, London

Cuff, E.C. and Payne, G.C.F. (eds) (1979) *Perspectives in Sociology*, Allen and Unwin, London

Delamont, S. (1980) *The Sociology of Women: An Introduction*, George Allen and Unwin, London

Denzin, N.K. (1977) *Sociological Methods*, McGraw–Hill, New York

Dingwall, R. (1977) *The Social Organisation of Health Visitor Training*, Croom Helm, London

Freeman, H.E., Levine, S. and Reeder, C.G. (eds) (1972) *Handbook for Medical Sociology*, 2nd edn, Prentice Hall, Englewood Cliffs

Garfinkel, H. (1967) *Studies in Ethnomethodology*, Prentice Hall, Englewood Cliffs

Goldthorpe, J. E. (1985) *An Introduction to Sociology*, 3rd edn, University Press, Cambridge

Kendall, P.L. and Reader, G.G. (1972) Contributions of sociology to medicine. In *Handbook for Medical Sociology*, 2nd edn, Prentice Hall, Englewood Cliffs

Leslie, G. R., Larson, R. F. and Gorman, B. L. (1980) *Introductory Sociology: Order and Change in Society*, 3rd edn, University Press, Oxford

Mechanic, D. (1968) *Medical Sociology: A Selective View*, Free Press, New York

Melia, K. (1986) Review essay: Imperialism, paternalism and the writing of introductory texts, *Sociology of Health and Illness*, 8(1), 86–98

Mills, C.W. (1959) *The Sociological Imagination*, Penguin, London

Murcott, A. (1989) Book review. *Sociology of Health and Illness*, II(1), 83–85

Payne, G., Dingwall, R., Payne, J. and Carter, M. (1981) *Sociology and Social Research*, Routledge and Kegan Paul, London

Perry, A. (1987) Sociology in the curriculum. In *The Curriculum in Nursing Education* (eds P.Allan and M.Jolley), Croom Helm, London, pp. 126–148

Seeley, J. (1966) The 'making' and 'taking' of problems. *Social Problems*, 14, 382–389

Silverman, D. (1981) Translator's Introduction, In Boudon, R. (1981) *The Logic of Social Actions*, Routledge, London

Smith, J. (1976) *Sociology and Nursing*, Churchill Livingstone, Edinburgh

Stacey, M. (1988) *The Sociology of Health and Healing*, Unwin Hyman, London

Theodore, J. (1989) Sociology by any other name. *Nursing Times*, 85(19), 74–75

Tuckett, D. and Kaufert, J.M. (eds) (1978) *Basic Readings in Medical Sociology*, Tavistock, London

United Kingdom Central Council for Nursing, Midwifery and Health Visiting (1986) *Project 2000: A New Preparation for Practice*, UKCC, London

Chapter 5

Social policy perspectives

Peter George

Although social policy is very important in the life of everyone living in modern Britain, and especially for anyone employed in one of the social services, most people would find it difficult to define. They might associate it with national insurance, income support or other benefits. They might think of services provided by local social services departments, such as social work, home helps or day centres for the elderly. They might recall debates about poverty or community care. These are indeed aspects of social policy, but there is much more to it than that. In the first section of this chapter, three different approaches to understanding social policy will be examined. Students may find in the literature that social policy is variously understood as policy for:

- The provision of social services
- The control or elimination of social problems
- Maintaining or changing social relationships.

Social policy and social services

This is the approach found in most textbooks of social policy (Brown, 1985; Rees, 1985; Young, 1985; Pascall, 1986; Hill, 1988). The social services referred to vary from one text to another but usually include social security, health services, employment services, housing, education and personal social services. Each of these may require a little explanation.

Social security refers to cash benefits like national insurance, income support, family credit, child benefit and housing benefit. Statutory sick and maternity pay are also usually included, although provided by employers. Government action which influences provision of equivalent benefits by employers and commercial insurance companies may also be considered. The benefits involved replace or supplement income from other sources for people who are retired, widowed, orphaned, sick, unemployed, disabled or considered to be unable to meet essential needs from other resources (Alcock, 1987).

Health services include policies for the promotion of health, prevention of illness, and treatment, care and rehabilitation of sick and disabled people. Although these are associated with the National Health Service in Britain it is important to consider policies for the provision of such services by employers, voluntary organizations, commercial companies and, informally, by relatives, friends and neighbours (Allsop, 1984).

Employment services help people find, prepare and train for jobs. In Britain, Job Centres, the Employment Training Scheme and Youth Training Scheme, and special employment services for disabled people are examples. Careers services provided in schools and colleges, private employment agencies and training services provided by employers might also be included (Lonsdale, 1985).

Housing policy generally refers to government action to influence the supply of housing, its quality, and people's access to it. These policies concern not only council housing but also owner-occupied and privately rented housing (Donnison and Ungerson, 1982).

Education, in the sense of policies for the provision of schools, colleges and universities, is usually included in discussions of social policy (Young, 1985 chapter 8; Hill, 1988, chapter 8), despite the fact that the study of educational services tends to have developed in relative isolation from other aspects of the welfare state. It is argued that education policies have always been a means of achieving social ends. Certainly, the 1944 Education Act, together with the National Insurance Act and the National Health Service Act, was regarded as one of the three pillars of the welfare state and governments since then have all regarded it as a vital instrument of social policy (Finch, 1984).

Personal social services include residential homes, day centres, domiciliary services and social work support and advice for old people, people who are physically or mentally impaired, children or anyone else in need of such social care. In Britain they may be associated with the Local Authority Social Services Departments but they may also be provided by voluntary and commercial suppliers and employers, and informally by families and friends and neighbours (Webb and Wistow, 1987).

While social policy, in this sense, means government social policy, it is not restricted to social services provided by government. Government policy may be that these services should be provided by employers, families, voluntary organizations and commercial suppliers as well as, or rather than, by the state. Indeed, one of the key areas of debate in social policy is about the part which these different agencies play and should play in the provision of social services.

Social policy and social problems

The provision of social services by government or other agencies is often regarded as a collective response to social problems or socially recognized needs. Thus social security may be seen as a response to people's need for some minimum income for subsistence or effective participation in society or a response to the problem of poverty. Health services can be regarded as a response to the problem of disease or to people's needs for health care. Employment services are one response to the problem of unemployment or to people's need for useful employment. Housing policies are a response to the problems of slums and homelessness or to people's needs for some minimum of shelter or a home. Education policies could be seen as a response to the problem of ignorance or to people's needs to acquire knowledge and skills for personal development, employment and citizenship. Finally, personal social services might be regarded as a response to fractured or strained relationships in families and communities, or to the needs of vulnerable people for social care.

In this approach the crucial questions in social policy have to do with the definition and measurement of social needs or problems and the determination of the most appropriate response to them. A good example is the long-term debate about the definition, measurement and explanation of poverty in Britain and about how best to provide for, or reduce, the numbers of poor people (Holman, 1978; Alcock, 1987). Another is the contemporary debate about the definition, measurement and explanation of inequalities in health and how best to reduce them (Townsend, Davidson and White-head, 1988).

This approach is certainly broader than a narrow concern with description and analysis of the social services which, from this perspective, are but one set of institutions through which poverty or illness can be ameliorated or reduced. Economic policies for full employment and incomes, the regulation of advertising, food and fuel policies, the regulation of working conditions and many other forms of government action might be seen as having a bearing on the reduction of poverty and illness. However, there are a number of difficulties with this approach. It is difficult to draw the boundaries between social policies and other policies which have an impact on social problems and social needs. It is difficult to define 'social problems' and 'social needs' independently from the social and political processes involved in creating policies to deal with them, so that the policies cannot be seen simply as a response to the needs and problems. On the contrary, it has been argued that 'needs' and 'problems' are socially constructed in the process of policy formation (Blumer, 1971). There is also evidence to suggest that needs and problems have little influence on the allocation of resources in the social services. For example, it has been suggested that an 'inverse care law' operates in the National Health Service, so that the greater the need for health care or the problems of illness in an area, the lower will be the quantity and quality of health services available and vice versa (Tudor Hart, 1971). Finally, it has been pointed out that defining social policies as a response to social needs and problems makes them seem more benign in intention than they sometimes are. The social policies of apartheid in South Africa, or the attempt to achieve Aryan purity and dominance in Nazi Germany, would not be regarded by many people as benign (Titmuss, 1974, p.26).

Social policy and social relationships

Apartheid and Nazi social policies involved attempts to establish and maintain the superiority of one race over another. Their focus was the structure of social relationships in those societies, and it might be argued that this is the focus of all social policies. Social policies are policies which are intended to maintain or change relationships between rich and poor, men and women, husbands and wives, parents and children, young and old, healthy and temporarily able-bodied and sick and disabled people, those who are employed and those who are not, and so on. These policies may: segregate or integrate; increase or reduce dependency and stigma; encourage or discourage caring, sharing, cooperation or mutual aid; sustain or diminish discrimination and oppression; increase or decrease inequalities in resources, opportunities or power. In this sense law and action relating to race relations, equal opportunities for men and women, marriage and divorce, the rights and obligations of parents and children, and the rights and obligations of employers and employees are all elements of a country's social policies as well as government action relating to social services and the latter is just one means government has of influencing social relationships. This approach to social policy can be found in the work of Townsend and Walker in Britain and Gil in the USA (Gil, 1973; Townsend, 1975; Walker, 1984).

When considering these and other approaches to social policy it is important to recognize that definitions of social policy are fraught with political implications. Narrower definitions are more likely to be suggested by writers who believe in minimum government action to protect a minority of the population who cannot provide or fend for themselves in a competitive society. The widest definitions appeal to those who regard social policy as a strategy for social reconstruction to create a more equal, fraternal and democratic society. In between are definitions which equate social policy with the provision of more or less universal social services in a social system which combines these elements of the welfare state with a market economy and political democracy. Like the definition of social policy, the investigation of social needs and problems and the design and implementation of social policies are the subject of moral and political arguments which combine facts and values. The production of knowledge in the field of social policy is thus deeply influenced by the values of the organizations, groups and individuals involved. The next section of this chapter is concerned with some aspects of the nature and uses of such knowledge.

Knowledge and social policy

Social policy studies fall into two broad, overlapping groups: investigations *of* social policy, and investigations *for* social policy.

Investigations of social policy

The investigation of social policy is a scholarly activity primar- ily concerned with understanding and explaining the nature, development and consequences of social policies, social legisla- tion and social welfare institutions, rather than with making a practical contribution to current development in social policy and the social services. The study of social policy has become an element in the education of many professions involved in the social services, for example social workers and health visitors. It is assumed that they need a knowledge of social policy to help their clients, to relate their own work to that of others involved with their clients, and because as responsible professionals they should play an informed part in debates about the future of social policy. It was partly the development of such teaching which led to the establishment of the study of social policy in higher education. (The first academic chair in the subject was established in 1950 at the London School of Economics). Teaching and research in social policy in this sense is concerned with: exploration and explanation of social needs and problems; analysis of the social and political pro- cesses through which such needs and problems are identified and action taken to deal with them; description and analysis of the social welfare policies, institutions and practices which emerge from such action; and critical appraisal of the impact of those policies, institutions and practices on individuals, groups and society. This can be illustrated by reference to studies of poverty and social security. These have involved studies of: the nature, extent and causes of poverty; the politics of poverty; the development of poor relief, social insurance, social assist- ance and other forms of provision for the poor, past and present; the effect of social security provision on people's standards of living and behaviour, and on the distribution of income or the level of employment in society (see Alcock, 1987, and the studies to which he refers: Donnison, 1982; Macgregor, 1981). Clearly, such studies could provide know- ledge which might influence policy makers even when that is not their primary purpose. Indeed, poverty research like that of Townsend (1979) might be regarded as 'strategic social sci- ence' concerned to explore concepts and test theories but with a focus on broad policy issues.

Rather different are comparative studies of the development of welfare states. This has been a growth area in the last decade (Castles, 1984; Jones, 1985). Many of these studies might be regarded as examples of 'basic social research' (Bulmer, 1978), concerned to explore concepts and models and test theories of the welfare state. Some of the theories in question regard the growth of welfare states as an inevitable consequence of industrialization or modernization, while others emphasize the role of class conflicts and social movements, and yet others the significance of ideologies and the pressure of vested interests from the beneficiaries and providers of the services. (For a critical introduction to such 'perspectives', see Williams, 1989.) Such studies may cast light on the limits of social reform, or provide arguments and evidence for those advocating particular policies, but they do not have a direct influence on social policy.

Different again are philosophical analyses of the moral and political ideas and principles on which social policies are based: ideas about needs, rights, justice, equality, democracy and participation, liberty, community, and so on. Such analyses can help to clarify concepts and arguments which are used in day to day political debates about health and welfare services, but are not necessarily linked to the promotion of particular policies (Plant, Lesser and Taylor-Gooby, 1980; Weale, 1983).

Investigations for social policy

The deliberate search for knowledge which will be useful in the process of developing specific social policies is the second broad category of studies. Three kinds of role may be played by social analysts and social researchers who are involved in this production of knowledge for social policy.

The first is intelligence and monitoring, that is the collection, presentation and analysis of statistics of social and economic trends, social expenditure and social service activities which may be used in formulating, justifying and evaluating social policies. There are many examples. Most people are aware of the population censuses which are conducted every ten years and of the recording of births, marriages and deaths. Death registrations are used to compile statistics on the causes of death in different 'social classes' and these are one source of evidence about trends in inequalities in health. The government Office of Population Censuses and Surveys also carries out regular surveys of social conditions like the General Household Survey. Many statistics are compiled using data recorded by government departments and social services during their daily activities. What is recorded and how it is recorded may be influenced by social scientists and government statisticians to make it more useful in formulating and monitoring social policies. It may also be influenced by governments anxious to present their policies in the best possible light. A good example of debates about the way statistics are collected by governments is the controversy about changes made in the collection of statistics about unemployment in Britain in the 1980s (Unemployment Unit, 1986, 1988). The statistics which are most useful to students of social policy are summarized annually in *Social Trends* (Central Statistical Office, 1988). Not all intelligence and monitoring is done by the government. Many interest groups and non-government organizations are also involved. One example is the annual report produced by the National Society for the Prevention of Cruelty to Children (NSPCC) on the statistics of child abuse. Another is the alternative statistics on unemployment produced by the Unemployment Unit. Some organizations have arisen from discontent with government information and seek to produce alternative data or alternative analyses of government statistics. For example, the work of the Radical Statistics Health Group might be of interest to nurses and other health workers (Radical Statistics Health Group, 1987).

The second kind of role is the investigation of a specific problem with a view to making practical suggestions about how to tackle it. Much research done by social scientists is of this kind. The work may be done 'independently' with the help of grants from research councils and foundations, or it may be done under contract for a government department or other agency. In the first case the researcher may have more freedom to define the problem and the methods of investigation, and to publish the findings, but more difficulty influencing policy makers. In the second, there is more direct access to policy makers but the agency defines the problem and the broad lines, if not the methods, of investigation and controls publication. Many examples of this kind of research are to be found among investigations of the numbers, living conditions and relationship to the social services of particular groups like disabled people (Glendinning, 1983; Martin and White, 1988; Office of Population Censuses and Surveys, 1988) or lone mothers (Millar, 1989). In the latter case the government's concern about the growing numbers of lone mothers dependent on social security led the Department of Social Security to commission a major survey of the dynamics of lone parents, and the Department of the Environment to commission a study of the housing consequences of relationship breakdown (Brad-shaw, 1989). Studies may be made of the delivery of services, such as the many studies of low take-up of social security benefit (for a review of these studies, see Deacon and Brad-shaw, 1983) or of preventative health care in pregnancy and early childhood (Dowling, 1983), and the many studies of residential care (Sinclair, 1988). These are just a few examples from a large volume of social policy research.

The third kind of research for policy is 'action research', in which action to implement policies is accompanied by re-search to appraise the results. Such research became popular with governments in Britain and the USA in the 1960s. The most prominent examples in Britain involved stimulating educational innovation in selected areas to reduce social and educational disadvantages amongst disadvantaged families, the so-called 'Educational Priority Area' projects, and the community development projects in which a variety of initia-tives were taken in selected areas of multiple deprivation to identify problems, establish development programmes and evaluate their success or failure (Halsey, 1972; Loney, 1983). More recently this kind of activity has been linked with attempts to find new and more effective ways of providing community care in a variety of projects around the country, like experiments with patch- or community-based social work (Hadley and McGrath, 1980; Beresford and Croft, 1986), and the provision of intensive community care to elderly people who would otherwise have been admitted to residential homes (Challis and Davies, 1986; Davies and Challis, 1986).

The role of policy research: problem solving and problem setting

Many accounts of the relationship between social research and social policy distinguish between pure and applied research but, as the two previous sections suggest, this is an oversimpli-fication, and it may be better to think in terms of a continuum, from basic research which may have future policy signific-ance, to action research which is embroiled in implementing and evaluating policy initiatives but has theoretical signific-ance (Bulmer, 1978).

The role of social research is commonly conceived to be to produce knowledge which can be used to solve problems. It has been argued that this 'problem solving image' is the dominant image of the relationship between social research and social policy (Schon, 1980; Rein, 1983). Research is thus seen as producing knowledge which helps to clarify problems, develop and appraise alternative solutions, and evaluate policies once they have been implemented. However, there have been several objections to this view of the role of research in social policy.

The first is that social research is seldom used in this way but is often used for other purposes, such as delaying decisions or providing a rationale for policies that have already been decided and programmes that have already been implemented (Weiss, 1978).

A second criticism of the 'problem solving' approach is that it treats the 'problem' as given. Yet there are no problems which exist independently of our efforts to deal with them. 'Social problems' are constructed by people in their attempts to explain and act on some aspect of their social world which they find disturbing. Social research is, then, part of this process of constructing the problem. Some social scientists have begun to analyse the social and political processes involved in the construction of 'social problems' (Blumer, 1971; Spector and Kitsuse, 1977). One good example of this kind of work in Britain is Parton's study of the 'politics' of child abuse (Parton, 1985). It can be argued that this problem did not exist until recently. This is not to deny that children were sometimes neglected or ill-treated by the adults who were caring for them. However, the 'battered child syndrome' was not identified until 1961 in the USA when Dr C. Henry Kemp ran a seminar on it at the annual meeting of the American Academy of Pediatricians. The choice of title for the seminar was itself important in gaining the attention of medical practitioners and the public and encouraging state action, not least because it emphasized the clinical rather than the criminal character of the problem. In Britain the 'battered baby syndrome' was a matter for discussion among forensic pathologists and paediatricians from 1963, but it was the work of the NSPCC Battered Baby Research Unit between 1968 and 1972 that first brought it to the attention of the media and a wider public. Then, in 1973, the death of Maria Caldwell and the ensuing public inquiry, against the background of growing concern about violence in society, and the interest of the Secretary of State for Health and Social Services, played a crucial part in establishing physical abuse of children as a social problem. Within a decade, baby and child battering was first to become 'non-accidental injury' and then 'child abuse' as neglect and mental and sexual abuse were added to the catalogue of concerns. These changes of the name of the problem in themselves indicate stages in its construction.

A third difficulty with the 'problem solving' view of knowledge in social policy is that attempted solutions to social problems often have unintended consequences which come to be perceived as problems in their own right. An example is the way in which high-rise flats, built as a solution to the problem of rehousing slum dwellers, later came to be regarded as a problem in themselves.

Finally, most problems which remain public issues for some time involve multiple goals which may be incompatible with each other. For example, it has been pointed out that there is probably no solution to the problem of providing an adequate income to reduce poverty while simultaneously maintaining incentives to work and keeping government spending down (Rein, 1976, p.56). If this is so, then a choice has to be made about which goal to optimize, and while the choice may be informed by knowledge, it cannot be made on the basis of knowledge alone.

For all these reasons it has been argued by Schon that 'the essential difficulties in social policy have more to do with problem setting than with problem solving' (Schon, 1980, p.255). The example he gives is of two different accounts of the problem of slums. In the first account, the slum is an area of overcrowded and decaying housing, inadequate streets and recreation facilities, with too few parks and open spaces and too little light and air. Its problems can be solved only by comprehensive demolition, replanning and rebuilding. The second account describes the slum as a community characterized by residential stability which attracts sentiments of attachment from its residents, not least because of the close social relationships among them. Demolition and rehousing will destroy the community and intensify the stresses experienced by the people who live in it. Schon calls these different accounts 'stories'. Each story selects different aspects of slum life for its main elements. In the first, these elements are 'decay', 'health', 'comprehensive planning' and 'reconstruction'. In the second they are 'community', 'spatial identity', 'informal social networks' and 'dislocation'. Each places the elements of its story in a different 'frame': of decay and reconstruction in the first account, and of communities, their threatened dissolution and their preservation in the second. Each story constructs a different view of social reality, and in the process makes a 'normative leap from data to recommendations, from facts to values, from is to ought' (Schon, 1980 p.265). Each story or account of the problem employs what Schon calls a 'generative metaphor'. In one case, the slum is like a disease to be cured; in the other, like a natural community to be protected or restored. Schon argues that such metaphors make the diagnosis and prescription of a solution for a social problem seem obvious. However, they may be misleading, and to avoid being misled it may be necessary to become aware of the metaphors which are shaping our perception of social problems so that we can subject them to critical scrutiny.

The trouble is that the metaphors underlying our accounts of social problems are usually tacit, so that we are completely unaware of them. Schon suggests that we can become critically aware of them only if our 'stories' are subjected to a critical analysis rather than literary criticism. When this is done, just as Schon does in the two conflicting accounts of slums, it often becomes clear that a debate about social policy poses a dilemma rather than a problem. That is to say, no available choice is a good one because the debate involves a conflict of ends which are incommensurable. In the example of the slums the choice appears to be between a healthier physical environment in which to live and the community which will be lost in the process of clearance and reconstruction. Such dilemmas can seldom be resolved by reference to facts, but Schon suggests that they may be resolved by constructing a new problem setting story containing elements drawn from the earlier stories. In the example of the slums, improvement, involving families and groups in the area in collaboration with each other and local government, may be the basis of such a new problem setting story. The role of local government in this story is to provide resources and expertise to enable families and groups to improve their own homes and local facilities, whilst itself taking on the task of improving services like roads and sewers.

Schon's example of conflicting accounts of slums is only one of many which might be taken from the field of social policy. Poverty has been regarded as a problem of culture, a way of life adapted to the experience of material deprivation on the margins of society. It has also been regarded as a problem of structure, of economic, social and political institutions which stack the odds against some people and in favour of others. Similarly, one account of the problem of inequality in health treats it as a consequence of differences in people's life-style and behaviour, and another as the outcome of material advantages and disadvantages in income, employment and living and working conditions.

Indeed, as was suggested in the first part of this chapter, there are conflicting accounts of the nature of social policy. One story is that it is about government-sponsored charity for the needy, another that it is about minimal entitlements for all citizens, and a third that it is about strategies to maintain or reconstruct social relationships and social institutions. What Schon's approach suggests is that these conflicting perspectives on social policy are unlikely to be reconciled by reference to knowledge alone. If indeed they can be reconciled, it will be through exposing and reflecting on the metaphors on which they are based so that new metaphors may be encouraged to emerge. Schon argues that this is a creative process which 'we are sometimes able to perform intuitively but which we cannot yet describe and model satisfactorily' (Schon, 1980, p.279).

Before leaving this section it is important to note that there is no suggestion that problem setting should *replace* problem solving in the production of knowledge for social policy, just that problem solving should be seen as a special case of social policy research, and not as the whole field of inquiry.

Conclusion

Social policy has much in common with nursing for it is not simply an object of systematic study but a field of practice. It is an object of study and a field of practice to which many disciplines contribute. Neither in nursing nor in social policy is it possible to separate moral issues from the study or the practice. In both, theories tend to combine values and explanations and their relationship to practice is problematic. As in nursing, knowledge in social policy is not produced only in universities and research institutes and then applied to practice. It also has to be developed in and through practice. Indeed, it has been suggested that practice-based research, conducted by practitioner-researchers, and producing empirically-based models of practice, could become the leading edge of new developments in social policy research and the social sciences (Rein, 1983). In this respect too, social policy and nursing may have something in common with each other.

References

Alcock, P. (1987) *Poverty and State Support*, Longman, London

Allsop, J. (1984) *Health Policy and the National Health Service*, Longman, London

Beresford, P. and Croft, S. (1986) *Whose Welfare: Private Care or Public Services*, Lewis Cohen Urban Studies Centre, Brighton

Blumer, H. (1971) Social problems as collective behaviour. *Social Problems*, **18(2)**, 298–306

Bradshaw, J. (1989) *Lone Parents: Policy in the Doldrums*, Family Policy Studies Centre, London

Brown, M. (1985) *Introduction to Social Administration in Britain*, 6th edn, Hutchinson, London

Bulmer, M. (1978) *Social Policy Research*, Macmillan, London

Castles, F. (1984) The welfare state in comparative perspective. In *Open University D355 Course Team, Social Policy and Social Welfare, Block 2, Unit 6*, Open University Press, Milton Keynes

Central Statistical Office (1988) *Social Trends 18*, HMSO, London

Challis, D. and Davies, B. (1986) *Case Management in Community Care: An Evaluated Experiment in the Home Care of the Elderly*, Gower, Aldershot

Davies, B. and Challis, D. (1986) *Matching Resources to Needs in Community Care*, Gower, Aldershot

Deacon, A. and Bradshaw, J. (1983) *Reserved for the Poor: the Means Test in British Social Policy*, Blackwell, Oxford

Donnison, D. (1982) *The Politics of Poverty*, Martin Robertson, Oxford

Donnison, D. and Ungerson, C. (1982) *Housing Policy*, Penguin, London

Dowling, S. (1983) *Health for a Change*, Child Poverty Action Group, London

Finch, J. (1984) *Education as Social Policy*, Longman, London

Gil, D. (1973) *Unravelling Social Policy*, Schenkman Publishing, Cambridge MA

Glendinning, C. (1983) *Unshared Care: Parents and their Disabled Children*, Routledge, London

Hadley, R. and McGrath, M. (eds) (1980) *Going Local: Neighbourhood Social Services*, Bedford Square Press, London

Halsey, A.H. (1972) *Educational Priority*, Vol. 1, HMSO, London

Hill, M. (1988) *Understanding Social Policy*, 3rd edn, Blackwell, Oxford

Holman, R. (1978) *Poverty: Explanations of Social Deprivation*, Martin Robertson, Oxford

Jones, C. (1985) *Patterns of Social Policy: An Introduction to Comparative Analysis*, Tavistock Press, London

Loney, M. (1983) *Community Against Government*, Heinemann, London

Lonsdale, S. (1985) *Work and Inequality*, Longman, London

Macgregor, S. (1981) *The Politics of Poverty*, Longman, London

Martin, J. and White, A. (1988) *The Financial Circumstances of Disabled Adults Living in Private Households*, OPCS Report 2, HMSO, London

Millar, J. (1989) *Poverty and the Lone Parent: the Challenge to Social Policy*, Avebury, Aldershot

Office of Population Censuses and Surveys (1988) *The Prevalence of Disability Among Adults: OPCS Surveys of Disability in Britain Report 1*, HMSO, London

Parton, N. (1985) *The Politics of Child Abuse*, Macmillan, London

Pascall, G. (1986) *Social Policy: A Feminist Analysis*, Tavistock Press, London

Plant, R., Lesser, H. and Taylor-Gooby, P. (1980) *Political Philosophy and Social Welfare: Essays on the Normative Basis of Welfare Provision*, Routledge, London

Radical Statistics Health Group (1987) *Facing the Figure*, Radical Statistics, London

Rees, A.M. (1985) *T.H. Marshal's Social Policy*, 5th edn, Hutchinson, London

Rein, M. (1976) *Social Science and Public Policy*, Penguin, London

Rein, M. (1983) *From Policy to Practice*, Macmillan, London

Schon, D. (1980) Generative metaphor: a perspective on problem-setting in social policy. In *Metaphor and Thought* (ed. A. Orton), Cambridge University Press, New York, pp. 254–283

Sinclair, I. (ed.) (1988) *Residential Care: The Research Reviewed*. Report of the Independent Review of Residential Care, Vol. 2, HMSO, London

Spector, M. and Kitsuse, J.I. (1977) *Constructing Social Problems*, Cummings, Menlo Park, CA, pp. 407–419

Titmuss, R. (1974) *Social Policy*, Allen and Unwin, London

Townsend, P. (1975) *Poverty in the United Kingdom*, Penguin, London

Townsend, P. (1979) *Sociology and Social Policy*, Penguin, London

Townsend, P., Davidson, N. and Whitehead, M. (1988) *Inequalities in Health*, Penguin, London

Tudor Hart, J. (1971) The inverse care law. *Lancet*, i, 405–412

Unemployment Unit (1986) *Unemployment Bulletin No. 22*

Unemployment Unit (1988) *Unemployment Bulletin No. 27*

Walker, A. (1984) *Social Planning*, Blackwell, Oxford

Weale, A. (1983) *Political Theory and Social Policy*, Macmillan, London

Webb, A. and Wistow, G. (1987) *Social Work, Social Care and Social Planning: the Personal Social Services since Seebohm*, Longman, London

Weiss, C.H. (1978) *Using Social Research for Public Policy-making*, Teakfield, Farnborough

Williams, F. (1989) *Social Policy: A Critical Introduction*, Polity Press, Oxford

Young, P. (1985) *Mastering Social Welfare*, Macmillan, London

Chapter 6

Psychological perspectives

Elisabeth Clark

This chapter aims to convey a realistic picture of what psychology is, discuss some of the tensions inherent in the study of human behaviour, and explore some of the difficulties that may arise when theoretical insights are borrowed from one discipline and applied to nursing.

Nurses and psychologists share a common area of concern. Psychology is concerned with understanding the experience and behaviour of the individual, while nurses are involved with caring for the individual. Increasingly, the emphasis in nursing is being placed on the maintenance of health rather than on treating illness and disease, and more people are being cared for in the community than in hospital. Such changes mean that nurses need to have a greater understanding of normal functioning and, more specifically, of ways of helping people to help themselves. This implies a knowledge of psychological processes. For instance, the factors which affect people's understanding and memory of important instructions and their compliance with instructions when not being supervised by others have been systematically investigated (e.g. Ley and Morris, 1984; Ley, 1988). This is an important area of concern for health education and for all those working to maintain the independence and well-being of people being cared for in the community.

A developing understanding of psychology should encourage practitioners to examine specific aspects of their own and other people's behaviour, and to challenge some of the unquestioned assumptions that are made about certain human experiences and behaviours. Psychological knowledge may also help nurses to understand themselves better as well as their patients/clients, and thus contribute to the scientific basis of health care.

Psychology is, however, just one of the disciplines that are concerned with the systematic study of people and their behaviour. Others include sociology, anthropology, economics and politics; they are all sometimes referred to collectively as the 'social sciences'. Psychology is specifically concerned with understanding the behaviour and experience of human beings, i.e. what makes people 'tick'. Psychologists investigate both *why* people do things and also *how* they do them. Any claim made by a psychologist about how or why people do things is usually backed by some kind of evidence, rather than by opinion or speculation.

In order to understand people better, psychologists have to deal with a diverse range of subject matter. As a consequence, psychology touches virtually every aspect of human activity and daily life and tackles questions such as:

- Can memory be improved?
- What methods of child-rearing produce well-adjusted adults?
- How do children learn to read?
- How can personality be accurately assessed?
- Is intelligence inherited or acquired through experience?

Psychologists have worked on, and continue to investigate, many interesting questions. The questions listed above are merely intended to provide an indication of the range of topics and questions that are studied by psychologists. The list of contents from any introductory psychology textbook (see, for example, Atkinson *et al.*, 1990) will also illustrate this breadth of study.

Perhaps not surprisingly this range of topics has necessitated the development of different approaches (sometimes referred to as 'schools') within the discipline. Psychologists do not approach their work in the same way and do not necessarily make the same assumptions about what should be studied, or even how it should be studied. In providing a realistic flavour of psychology, it is necessary, therefore, to consider some of the very real tensions and differences that exist within a discipline that sets out to describe and explain human behaviour and experience. In fact, one of the strengths of psychology may be that it has not adopted a single unified approach to the study of behaviour and experience. As we shall see, different approaches have developed and have provided different kinds of insight into the subject matter.

An example will help to illustrate how a specific behaviour might be studied and explained in different ways. Imagine a person is waiting at a pelican crossing on a busy road and then decides that it is safe and begins to walk across the road. This act of crossing a road may be described in a number of different ways:

- A response to the stimulus of a green light and a bleeping sound.
- Nerves activating the muscles that enable one to walk across the road.
- The decisions that enable the person to cross a busy road safely.
- Part of a plan to achieve a particular goal (such as walking to work, visiting a friend, etc.).

These descriptions illustrate the idea that any action, however simple, may be explained from several different points of view. Likewise, psychologists often study different aspects of a complex behaviour. The background and theoretical beliefs of a researcher will influence the research done and how findings are interpreted and reported. There is no single 'right' or 'wrong' approach in psychology, and the different approaches are certainly not mutually exclusive. Adequate explanation of any psychological phenomenon often requires a synthesis of several different approaches. In the next section five major approaches will be briefly outlined.

Psychophysiological approach

The psychophysiological approach aims to monitor physiological changes that accompany psychological events; for instance, the heart rate of most people will increase markedly under conditions of psychological, as well as physical stress. It seeks to identify the relationship between physiological processes and various aspects of behaviour. Psychophysiologists have studied a number of physiological changes including skin conductivity (known as the galvanic skin response), muscle tension, blood flow in various parts of the body, hormonal level in the bloodstream and electrical activity in the brain. Their research typically involves the use of highly sophisticated electronic measuring equipment in order to record specific

physiological responses accurately. Psychophysiological techniques have, for example, been used to investigate the effectiveness of meditation as a technique for inducing relaxation
and reducing physiological arousal (see Shapiro, 1985). However, due to the difficulties of undertaking psychophysiological
research, current knowledge and understanding of the relationships between specific behaviours and experiences and
neural functioning are still very limited.

Behavioural approach

This school emerged shortly after the turn of the twentieth
century and has dominated psychological research for many
years. Watson (1913) argued that psychology could only
become truly objective if it limited itself to the study of
behaviour (which is public) as opposed to consciousness
(which is private). Thus, within a behavioural approach,
psychologists primarily focus on the study of observable behaviour which is open to public inspection like the data of any
other natural science. Considerable emphasis is placed on
scientific rigour, objectivity and use of the experimental
method under tightly controlled conditions to study cause and
effect and produce general laws of behaviour.
   A strictly behavioural approach (known as radical be-
haviourism) limits itself to precise measurement of observable
events and overlooks all mental processes, since these cannot
be directly observed. Instead, behaviourists have tended to
focus on ways in which both animal and human behaviour is
influenced by the environment. This approach is sometimes
referred to as stimulus–response (S–R) psychology since behaviourists are mainly concerned with studying the antecedents
and consequences of specific behaviours. Knowledge of the
antecedents of a particular behaviour may enable us to
predict, and perhaps also to control, that behaviour. The term
'black box' has been used to acknowledge a link in the chain
between stimulus and response: a link which might enable
psychologists to explain the relationship between the two by
investigating the internal biochemical and mental processes
that occur between the reception of a stimulus and the
production of a response to that stimulus. Early behaviourists,
such as Watson, have been criticized for overlooking the
internal processes occurring within the 'black box'. Subsequently, a number of psychologists (who became known as

neo-behaviourists) chose to 'open the box' and acknowledge the existence of mental processes occurring between stimulus and response (see, for example, Tolman, Ritchie and Kalish, 1946).

Overall, behaviourists have made a substantial contribution to our understanding of behaviour; their behavioural principles are widely used in a number of different areas, including behaviour therapy, education and child psychology. Behavioural principles have, for instance, been successfully applied in the clinical field. Behaviourists assume that any behaviour which requires alteration (so-called maladaptive behaviour) is learned. Behaviour therapy can, therefore, be seen as a process of relearning. In order to do this, detailed information is needed about the frequency of the maladaptive behaviour (such as episodes of screaming), any situational triggers, and any reactions that may be reinforcing the behaviour. Using this information, a training programme may be designed which enables the maladaptive behaviour to be extinguished and a more appropriate behaviour to be substituted in its place.

Psychoanalytic approach

At about the same time as the behavioural approach was being developed in the United States, a very different approach was evolving in Europe. Freud (1856–1939) was initially responsible for developing the psychoanalytic approach based on his case studies of individual clients, and is regarded by some as the founder of modern psychology. As a qualified doctor, Freud studied the human mind and attempted to understand mental disorders that could not be explained from a purely physiological perspective. Freud's approach rested on the assumption that much of human behaviour is determined by unconscious processes, thoughts, fears and wishes that the person is unaware of and yet which influence behaviour. He claimed that people shut away, or repressed, conflicts in their lives, particularly ones occurring in childhood, because they were too painful to bear. Problems, such as anxiety or depression, arising in adulthood were assumed to be traceable to those conflicts that remained unresolved in the person's unconscious. Freud also believed that unconscious impulses could express themselves through slips of the tongue (so-called Freudian slips), mannerisms and dreams, in addition to the neurotic disorders mentioned above. Freudian emphasis on the unconscious and on inner life is clearly different from that of the behavioural approach with its focus on observable behaviour.

It is interesting to note that of all the psychological approaches, the psychoanalytic one would appear to have had the greatest impact on the general public. Berger (1965) highlights how many of the concepts of psychoanalytic theory, such as 'the unconscious', 'repression', and 'Freudian slips', have become part of our everyday language, and are often used without any understanding of their original context. Yet from within psychology, the psychoanalytic approach has perhaps been the focus of more debate than any other approach.

Humanistic approach

Meanwhile, there was mounting dissatisfaction in certain quarters with the widespread application of the experimental method to the study of human behaviour and development. The preoccupation with scientific rigour, objectivity and with explaining behaviour through general laws of cause and effect meant that many of the important aspects of human experience that distinguished human beings from other animals, including self-awareness, self-determination and individuality, could not be studied and had to be overlooked.

Thus, the humanistic approach emerged in the 1950s as a reaction to both the behaviourist and psychoanalytic traditions which were well established at the time. Consequently, it is sometimes referred to as the 'third force'. The founders of this movement, George Kelly, Carl Rogers and Abraham Maslow, firmly rejected any positivist approach that treats people as if they were objects to be manipulated by an experimenter, on the grounds that the task of understanding people and explaining their behaviour required different methods from those used by natural scientists to generate laws explaining the physical world.

A central concept in humanistic psychology is that of 'self', which refers to the set of beliefs a person holds about who and what he or she is, and the development of self – what is sometimes called our 'self-image'. They have chosen to focus on people's experience: their individual view of themselves and their world, and their interpretation of events, rather than on their behaviour *per se*. It seeks to understand events as they are experienced by the individual, and differs from the other approaches in the value it attaches to people's subjective experiences. Humanistic psychologists would argue that an individual's own view of his or her world is reality to the person concerned.

Humanistic psychologists place considerable emphasis on people's ability to make choices, consciously direct their own lives and take responsibility for their own actions. By contrast, both psychoanalytic and behaviourist approaches have tended to view people's behaviour as determined by forces outside of their control and play down the contribution of 'free will'. Thus, humanistic psychologists recognize that two people may act in the same way but for totally different reasons, or alternatively, may react very differently to the same situation. They claim that in order to understand human behaviour more fully it is necessary to study people's lives and experiences: their self-awareness, their feelings of self-esteem and their concept of themselves. Perhaps not surprisingly, some psychologists have been quick to dismiss such attempts to study 'inner life' as unscientific, particularly because the use of tightly controlled experiments to generate data is not considered to be either appropriate or desirable by the humanistic psychologist.

Cognitive approach

Whilst many psychologists largely choose to ignore what goes on within the organism between the reception of an external stimulus and a response to it, cognitive psychologists make this the major focus of their study. They argue that the brain actively processes the information it receives, rather than being a passive receptor of stimuli. The term 'cognition' refers to all conscious mental processes: perception, memory, attention, thinking, problem solving, imagination, reasoning, etc. To a cognitive psychologist, mental events and processes occurring within the person are considered to be as important as external stimuli for understanding behaviour. The systematic investigation of these higher mental processes began in its own right in the 1960s.

A cognitive approach may, therefore, be seen as complementary to a behavioural approach, since it attempts to open up and understand the 'black box' between a stimulus being received and the subsequent response to it. Implicit in much of the work of cognitive psychologists is the assumption that people are basically rational, reasoning beings, unlike those working within a psychoanalytic tradition who are primarily concerned with trying to understand people's more irrational behaviours.

Irrespective of approach, all psychologists attempt to make their answers to research questions as full and as objective as circumstances and current methodology permit. Psychology has certainly not yet arrived at a stage in its own development where insights from any particular approach can be dismissed as unimportant:

> The relationship between mind, brain and social context is the most complex which scientists are trying to tackle. It would be folly at this stage in our understanding to seek to restrict psychological science to particular styles of theory or method, or to particular aspects of human behaviour (British Psychological Society, 1988).

Conflict or synthesis?

So far, then, we have seen that 'psychology' has meant, and continues to mean, different things to different people. This should not come as any surprise; after all, it is difficult to get a group of nurses to agree on the definition of 'nursing'. Some people might argue that the existence of different approaches means that in reality nothing is known, that there are no 'hard' facts, and that anybody's guess is as good as any other person's. Alternatively, one could argue that the strengths of such diversity and the understanding gained from differing perspectives can be complementary, and may, therefore, be viewed as a positive rather than a negative quality of the discipline.

Social scientists often argue that human behaviour in its social context is so complex that no one view can provide an adequate explanation. Taking the example of the study of aggression, it is possible to identify the different ways in which it might be studied within each of the five approaches that have been discussed. A psychophysiologist would be likely to search for the parts of the brain that are responsible for, or trigger, aggressive behaviour. A behaviourist, on the other hand, would probably be more concerned with identifying particular environmental stimuli that provoke an aggressive outburst. A psychoanalyst might choose to investigate child-hood experiences and repressed conflicts as the key to under-standing aggressive outbursts. A humanistic psychologist is likely to explore individuals' perceptions of themselves, their experiences of aggression and the interpretation that they place on particular behaviours. Finally, a cognitive psycholo-gist might study how people represent certain events, relating to anger, in their minds and how different types of information might alter these mental representations. The most complete understanding of aggression can only be gained by combining the insights that emerge from these differing approaches. One of these approaches standing alone would only provide a partial explanation of a complex phenomenon such as aggres-sion.

Not every topic studied by psychologists, however, is studied from all five perspectives. Certain topics can only be invest-igated within specific approaches. For instance, personal growth and self-fulfilment are only studied by psychologists working within the humanistic tradition. Thus, the topic under investigation will determine the approach that is used. Some approaches are obviously more suited to a specific subject than others: a behavioural psychologist would not contemplate the study of unconscious processes, whilst a psychologist working within the psychoanalytic tradition would not study animal learning.

In order to distinguish clearly between them, the description above of the five different approaches places too great an emphasis on the differences between them. In practice, psy-chologists rarely confine themselves to a single school of thought, e.g. strictly behavioural or purely cognitive. Few researchers would wish to argue that one approach was able to provide the 'whole truth'. Most tend to be eclectic, that is to say, they draw from a number of approaches, depending on the topic that they are investigating. (See Chapman and Jones (1980) for an interesting description of how a number of leading British psychologists view their contribution to the discipline.)

Person and process perspectives

Psychological research may also be considered according to two further perspectives which cut across the five approaches that have been discussed. These have been referred to as the 'person' and 'process' perspectives (Greene, 1981).

The 'person' perspective is concerned with studying people as individuals, each with a unique blend of personality and experience. Thus, the major focus is the understanding of individual differences between people and how these differences affect behaviour. The 'process' perspective, on the other hand, does not attempt to study people as whole persons. Instead, it assumes that behaviour can best be explained by investigating the psychological processes which underlie basic human activities. Furthermore, these processes, such as memory, thinking and problem solving, tend to be studied in isolation. This perspective also assumes that these basic processes are universal to all humans. In this way, similarities rather than differences are investigated and emphasized

These two perspectives, therefore, highlight a further tension within psychology. Should psychology attempt to produce general laws of behaviour which apply universally, such as behavioural and cognitive psychologists aim to provide, or should psychologists treat people as individuals with their own unique blend of personality and experience, as advocated by humanistic psychologists? In contrast to the universal laws of the natural sciences which enable us to predict what will happen in certain well-defined circumstances, psychological findings may always be limited by their social and cultural context, and by the era in which they occur. Perhaps there are unlikely to be immutable laws of human behaviour.

It should be clear from the preceding discussion that the term 'psychology' covers a diversity of approaches with differing objectives. Indeed, Beloff (1973) argued that there is no such thing as a single discipline called psychology, but rather a collection of 'psychological sciences', each with its own focus and methods of study. More recently, the Working Party on the *Future of the Psychological Sciences*, commissioned by the British Psychological Society (1988), also adopted a catholic definition of psychology:

> in which a variety of approaches, if systematically pursued, and if open to rigorous criticism and challenge, are legitimate means of increasing our understanding. Orderly theorizing, systematic observation and measurement, and honest and careful interpretation and reporting of research findings are the hallmarks of the true discipline of psychological science.

Without a number of different approaches, the breadth of psychological thinking would necessarily be severely limited. Irrespective of the differences between the various approaches, they all aim to investigate aspects of behaviour and experience systematically, and adopt the individual as the major focus of study.

You may have noticed the use of the word 'systematic' in the previous paragraph. Few people would wish to disagree with the assertion that the research methods used by psychologists are systematic. So, for example, humanistic psychologists strive to investigate and describe subjective experience in an orderly way. There is, however, considerable disagreement among psychologists about what constitutes legitimate data. Not all psychologists are prepared to accept private experience (that is to say, an individual's personal account of conscious experience which cannot be independently verified) as legitimate data. Closely related to this, there is also a continuing debate about whether or not psychology is, or even should be, a science.

A basic claim of any scientific study is that of objectivity. But for obvious reasons the issue of objectivity creates challenges when human beings, with all their personal biases and assumptions, study fellow humans. Gahagan (1984) comments:

> ... amongst scientists students of human behaviour have a unique relationship with subject matter ... psychologists know (though in the past they have tried to pretend otherwise) that in essential respects they are the same as those whom they study. Furthermore, they are obliged to participate in the very processes they are attempting to objectify. For to study their subjects they have to interact with them, and whatever they 'find' will be a product of their own activities and processes as well as those of their subjects.

Scientific research aims to make statements which are regarded as true according to criteria that are public and which can be independently verified. Considerable emphasis is placed on objectivity and replicability. This raises the key issue of the usefulness of applying the same kind of narrow scientific standards to the study of humans as are applied to the investigation of natural events.

To have as its prime goal the attainment of scientific respectability and rigour as defined above, psychology would have to restrict its focus of study and abandon areas that are both interesting and important, including the study of human experience. The way in which individuals react to what they experience is by its very nature a 'private' matter; it cannot be directly observed and is not, therefore, open to public scrutiny. At present, psychologists do not have available research techniques which would enable them to study subjective experience in a manner that would satisfy strict scientific criteria.

Unless one modifies the strictly scientific approach (based on a natural sciences model of science), the study of human experience would have to be discontinued. On the other hand, if one accepts the desirability of studying these more subjective, but nonetheless important areas of human nature, then careful thought has to be given to the criteria that would be used to evaluate this work. The contribution of, say, humanistic psychologists studying aspects of experience would undoubtedly be dismissed as 'unscientific', and presumably rejected, if the narrow scientific criteria of validity alone were adopted.

Alternatively, the specific goals and assumptions of humanistic psychology could be used instead. Whilst humanistic psychologists themselves would see the latter as appropriate, it is important to recognize that in accepting such a position, one is rejecting the narrow view of psychology as a science modelled on the natural sciences. In consequence, any change in the criteria used for evaluation would need to be explicitly acknowledged and accepted as being appropriate.

Psychology and nursing

If nurses are to use knowledge from other disciplines, such as psychology, it is crucial that they should do so in an informed way, guided by a clear understanding of the different ways in which data may be collected and interpreted by researchers. The temptation to embrace ideas and theories from another discipline without careful consideration of either their contribution to that discipline or their contribution to nursing must be resisted. The next section, which focuses on some of the work undertaken by Maslow, illustrates some of the complexities of the relationship between psychological theory and nursing practice. It is noticeable that Maslow presents more hunches and hypotheses than empirical evidence. His research also provides insight into some of the very real methodological difficulties of studying human experience.

Maslow's theory of human motivation

Any theory referring to human needs is likely to appeal to health care practitioners. It is, however, necessary to go beyond intuitive reactions and examine the basis of the theoretical ideas in order to evaluate in an informed way their potential contribution to professional practice.

Abraham Maslow (1908–1970) was one of the founders of humanistic psychology. Four key assumptions about the nature of people underlie the work of all humanistic psychologists. When thinking about these assumptions it may be helpful to remember that they emerged out of the North American ideology of individualism and liberalism of the 1950s and 1960s. Against this political context, it is hardly surprising that considerable emphasis was placed on:

- The whole person rather than individual psychological processes in isolation.
- A person's conscious awareness of his or her own existence as distinct from that of other people (an existential perspective).
- The way in which an individual experiences and interprets his or her world (a phenomenological perspective).
- One's freedom to make choices and decisions and thus direct one's own actions.

These basic assumptions set humanistic psychology apart from other approaches in psychology. Humanistic psychologists have their own agenda. Their main aim is to help people explore and realize their potential as individuals, rather than generate specific theories of human behaviour. This aim has brought with it new methods and procedures. Since few of the topics of interest to humanistic psychologists lend themselves to either precise measurement or investigation in a laboratory, little use is made of experimental techniques or the statistical analysis of quantitative data. Instead, introspective accounts and interviews are frequently used to provide the basis of descriptions of people's conscious awareness. Ideally, an introspective account would communicate all the nuances of a person's flow of consciousness as they are experiencing it. In reality, however, such accounts tend to interfere with the experience itself and are recalled after the event, with all the problems associated with any retrospective data.

One of Maslow's prime concerns was to attempt to describe the characteristics of the so-called 'psychologically healthy person'. He adopted a positive and optimistic view of human nature, emphasizing people's desire for personal growth and self-fulfilment. Needless to say, his approach was markedly different from that of Freud, whose theory of human nature was almost entirely based on clinical work with patients suffering from some kind of emotional disturbance. By contrast, Maslow stressed the potential for personal growth in adulthood towards self-actualization, which he described as 'the full use and exploitation of talents, capacities, potentialities, etc.' in order 'to become everything that one is capable of becoming' (Maslow, 1987). Such an emphasis is almost certainly linked to North American self-confidence of the 1950s.

Thus, Maslow was concerned not only with how people are, but more importantly, with what people can become through continuing personal development during adulthood. There are three aspects of his work that are worthy of mention: a theory of motivation based on his well-known hierarchy of human needs; a description of the characteristics of self-actualizing people (self-actualization being the culmination of development in Maslow's hierarchy of needs), and his study of 'peak experiences'.

First, we shall consider Maslow's ideas on personal growth and motivation. Motivation is not an easy concept to define. It refers to the 'why' behind people's actions; a driving force which energizes behaviour – a process involving the experiencing of needs and their satisfaction. For example, a person who is thirsty (drive) is motivated to find something to drink (behaviour); a person who is ambitious (drive) works hard (behaviour).

When thinking about motives it soon becomes apparent that different people have differing motives for doing the same thing. Or, again, we find that an individual may have a range of motives for doing something, and some of these may not be obvious. For instance, what are your motives for reading this particular chapter? As a result of studying different kinds of motives in a range of situations, Maslow argued that motives could be classified, and that these categories could be arranged in a hierarchy from the most basic biological requirements necessary for survival to the expression of more complex psychological needs that become important only after more basic needs have been satisfied (Figure 6.1).

However, Maslow's classification introduces a further refinement: he made an important distinction between two

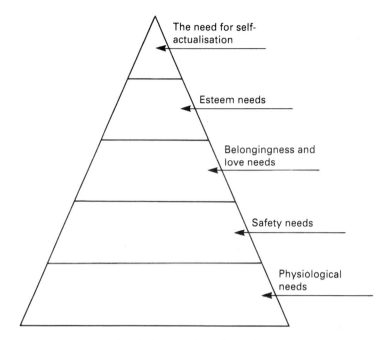

Figure 6.1   Maslow's hierarchy of needs

different types of motivation, growth motivation and deficiency motivation. We will start by looking at the latter, since deficiency motives are likely to be more familiar. The example of thirst presented above is based on the principle of deficiency motives: when a person is thirsty he or she drinks in order to remove, or at least reduce, the 'tension' caused by the deficiency; after drinking the motive disappears and equilibrium returns until next time. Although this approach (also referred to as the 'tension reduction' model of motivation) was based on work with animals, it can also apply to certain motives in humans, including thirst, hunger, temperature and tiredness.

Despite its widespread acceptance, a deficiency model is unable to account for the diversity and complexity of human behaviour. How would it explain doing something merely 'for the fun of it', for example? Maslow postulated growth motives to account for doing things even when there is no obvious need or deficiency. Thus, according to Maslow, humans are motivated not only to correct deficiencies but also to develop and grow and seek new experiences. If, however, a person is unable to fulfil, for whatever reason, the lower levels of need, this will prevent the development of individual potential reflected in the higher order needs.

In Figure 6.1, the first four levels are described by Maslow as deficiency needs which we are motivated to reduce in order to achieve a state of satisfaction. The expression of self-actualization, on the other hand, is an end in itself and is a growth need. Thus, Maslow's theory of motivation incorporates the notion of an 'end point' of development (self-actualization) as well as the process by which people move towards it. A necessary precondition for self-actualization is the satisfaction of deficiency needs; that is to say, you cannot move on before deficiency needs have at least partly been satisfied.

Maslow (1987) identified the characteristics of self-actualizers. He based this analysis on the study of a group of 49 people whom he admired and who were probably self-actualizers. Amongst this number were personal acquaintances and friends, public figures and exceptional people from the past, such as Einstein and the psychologist William James. He examined biographical information, and questioned friends/relatives and, wherever possible, the people themselves. According to Maslow, such people shared a number of characteristics including: creativity; spontaneity in thought and behaviour; good sense of humour; accurate perception of reality; refusal to be bound by convention; capacity for deep appreciation of basic experiences of life; acceptance of themselves and of others; ability to establish deep, satisfying relationships with a few, rather than many, people. They were also likely to have had what Maslow termed 'peak experiences': that is, a sudden heightening of consciousness – a 'state of being' characterized by an overwhelming feeling of wholeness, contentment, aliveness and delight; a transient moment of self-actualization. In addition, some negative tendencies were identified, including stubborness and a tendency to be ruthless. Since most of Maslow's sample who were still living were over the age of 60, he also suggested that self-actualization was associated with maturity.

There are, however, methodological flaws in the way this analysis was carried out. First, Maslow's sample was both highly selective and very limited in size. Second, many of the attributes are difficult to assess reliably. Third, he does not compare the self-actualizers with any other group of subjects. Fourth, some of the identified characteristics merely reflect attributes which determined their inclusion in the sample in the first place. Finally, his selection of attributes was almost certainly influenced by the North American culture of the era (the 1950s and 1960s). As Sugarman (1986) points out: 'Other cultures and other historical epochs may well challenge such an individually based definition of optimum human functioning (self-actualization) . . . A different end point might be achievable through a different route.'

Maslow's hierarchy of needs as presented in Figure 6.1, and in most other textbooks, suggests a fixed ordering of the different levels of need. This analysis reflects what he found to be the case for the majority of individuals in his study. He did, however, recognize a number of significant exceptions (Maslow, 1987). For instance, some people considered self-esteem to be more important than love – a reversal in levels three and four of the hierarchy. Maslow also recognized that in some highly creative people their need to create may take precedence over all their other needs. Thus, Maslow did *not* claim that his hierarchy of needs was either inevitable or universal, in spite of what others may have implied since.

One aspect of conscious experience of particular interest to Maslow was the 'peak experience' (PE) mentioned earlier. Maslow reported that those people whom he regarded as being psychologically healthy were especially likely to have PEs; he regarded such states as both a consequence of, and a means of achieving, optimal psychological development. However, Maslow's own account of PEs includes little evidence for the claims he made. Clearly it is difficult to investigate and describe complex and spontaneous experiential states in sufficient detail to enable others to distinguish a PE from other shifts in conscious experience reliably. Language may not provide a suitable means of communicating the necessary shades of conscious awareness. As Stevens (1990) concludes:

> We have, in effect, to take on trust or use our own life experience to confirm the conclusions he draws from his studies. Their value, however, is not as established facts, but lies in their capacity to stimulate us to think about our own experience, the way we live our lives and the alternatives open to us.

Such an outcome is very different from an informed evaluation of empirical data using agreed scientific criteria.

Many psychologists would acknowledge the desirability of recognizing individual differences between people and of studying the more subjective but none the less important aspects of human life. However, crucial differences are apparent in their reaction to this challenge. You may recall that early behaviourists chose to reject substantial areas of study simply because the key processes of 'mental life' could not be directly observed or measured. In contrast, humanistic psychologists have not restricted themselves to such a limited vision of what is possible. They remain, as the work of Maslow illustrates, determined to pursue new ways of studying experience.

While recognizing the continuing need to search for public and objective indicators of subjective states, Maslow (1968) made good use of people's capacity to reflect on conscious experience. He wrote:

> Nor ought we neglect the subjective data that we do have. It is unfortunate that we cannot ask a rat to give subjective reports. Fortunately, however, we can ask the human being, and there is no reason in the world why we should refrain from doing so until we have a better source of data.

Extracts such as this illustrate Maslow's open mindedness as to acceptable methods and his commitment to investigate previously unexplored yet important aspects of human behaviour.

Nevertheless, it is important to realize that many of Maslow's concepts have not been precisely defined and that his theories have not been sufficiently rigorously expressed to be testable. Consequently, empirical evidence is not available to support many of his assertions. Moreover, there are several instances in Maslow's own writing which make it clear that he was perfectly aware of the shortcomings of his work; he even cautioned about the use and validity of his theory:

> This book, like my previous one, is full of affirmations which are based on pilot researches, bits of evidence, on personal observation, on theoretical deduction and on sheer hunch ... they are hypotheses, i.e. presented for testing rather than for final belief. (Maslow, 1968) ...

> I of all people should know just how shaky this foundation [for his theory of motivation] is as a final foundation ... There are many things wrong with the sampling, so many in fact that it must be considered to be, in the classical sense anyway, a bad or poor or inadequate experiment, I am quite willing to concede it – because I'm a little worried about this stuff which I consider to be tentative being swallowed whole by all sorts of

enthusiastic people, who really should be a little more tentative in the way I am. (Maslow, 1965)

Despite this, the suggestion is frequently made that Maslow's hierarchy of needs might be used as a tool to assess patients' needs. The extract below illustrates the way in which Maslow's theory has been presented; it is taken from a discussion by the authors (Roper, Logan and Tierney, 1983) of their 'Activities of Living' model for nursing. They write:

> The priority which some ALs (activities of living) have over others is reflected in theories of human needs, for example, the analysis . . . by Abraham Maslow (1970). . . . The usual way of illustrating the hierarchy of human needs is by drawing a pyramid to infer the order of priority, those in the lowest category requiring to be at least minimally fulfilled before motivation is established to seek fulfilment of needs in the second category, and so on. Occasionally, as may happen during illness, the higher order needs may be submerged or engulfed by lower ones. As an example, after a serious accident, fulfilment of physiological and safety needs becomes of paramount importance and submerges all others. This example helps to establish that consideration of current priority of an individual's needs is an important part of the concept of basic human needs.

Knowing the background of Maslow's work raises a number of issues relating to the extrapolation of Maslow's findings; for example, how does it apply to people who are ill; can it be assumed that the theory applies irrespective of cultural background? His theory may make intuitive sense to individuals who come from a similar background, with its emphasis on achievement, individualism and materialism. However, it is questionable whether it pays sufficient attention to the fact that motives reflect both biological and social–cultural influences and the interaction between them.

The example of Maslow's hierarchy of needs and its widespread adoption within nursing highlights a number of important issues which apply to all psychological knowledge. Before 'borrowing' any set of theoretical ideas from any discipline, it is clearly necessary to be aware of the context and background of the research and the details of the original work; one cannot simply rely on second-hand accounts. Only after critically evaluating the research can one make an informed choice regarding the appropriateness or otherwise of adopting the theory in a nursing context. However tempting it might seem, this process of evaluation must not be short circuited. Once adopted, it is also necessary to evaluate a particular theory to verify its potential usefulness in practice.

Finally, it is important to recognize that although psychological knowledge is never prescriptive and will not provide 'recipes' for ensuring particular outcomes for practice, it can inform nursing judgement. Any clinical decision or action needs not only to take account of any relevant psychological evidence, but also the unique nature of the particular situation and the individual(s) concerned.

References

Atkinson, R.L., Atkinson, R.C., Smith, E.E., Bem, D.J. and Hilgard, E.R. (1990) *Introduction to Psychology* 10th edn, Harcourt Brace Jovanovich, San Diego

Beloff, J. (1973) *Psychological Sciences: A Review of Modern Psychology*, Lockwood Staples, Crosby

Berger, P.L. (1965) Towards a sociological understanding of psychoanalysis. *Social Research*, **32**, 26–41

British Psychological Society (1988) *The Future of the Psychological Sciences: Horizons and Opportunities for British Psychology*, BPS, London

Chapman, A. and Jones, D.M. (eds) (1980) *Models of Man*, British Psychological Society, London

Gahagan, J. (1984) *Social Interaction and its Management*, Methuen, London

Greene, J. (1981) *What is Psychology?* Unit 1 of Course DS262: Introduction to Psychology, Open University Press, Milton Keynes

Ley, P. and Morris, L. (1984) Psychological aspects of written information for patients. In *Contributions to Medical Psychology 3* (ed. S. Rachman), Pergamon, Oxford

Ley, P. (1988) *Communicating with Patients: Improving Communication, Satisfaction and Compliance*, Chapman and Hall, London

Maslow, A.H. (1965) *Eupsychian Management: A Journal*, Irwin-Dorsey, Homewood

Maslow, A.H. (1968) *Toward a Psychology of Being*, 2nd edn, Van Nostrand Reinhold, New York

Maslow, A.H. (1987) *Motivation and Personality*, 3rd edn, Harper and Row, New York

Roper, N., Logan, W.W. and Tierney, A.J. (eds) (1983) *Using a Model for Nursing*, Churchill Livingstone, Edinburgh

Shapiro, D.H. (1985) Clinical use of meditation as a self-regulating strategy: comments on Holmes' 1984 conclusions and implications. *American Psychologist*, **40**, 719–722

Stevens, R. (1990) Humanistic psychology. In *Introduction to Psychology*, Vol.1, (ed. I. Roth), Lawrence Erlbaum Associates in association with the Open University, Milton Keynes, pp. 417–469

Sugarman, L. (1986) *Life-span Development: Concepts, Theories and Interventions*, Methuen, London

Tolman, E.C., Ritchie, B.F. and Kalish, D. (1946) Studies in spatial learning: II. Place learning versus response learning. *Journal of Experimental Psychology*, **36**, 221–229

Watson, J.B. (1913) Psychology as the behaviourist sees it. *Psychological Review*, **20**, 158–177

Chapter 7

Moral perspectives*

David Cook

With the growing professionalization of nurses, both in terms of education and responsibility, questions about key moral issues have emerged; these are at both the intra- and inter-professional level. Inevitably, many of these questions coincide with those of medical colleagues, but the nursing profession is clear that the nurse's role with regard to patients is not exactly the same as that of the doctor. While sharing in the care of patients, the definition of 'care' is wider, not merely in terms of relationships but also in terms of acting on the patient's behalf as an advocate in settings where the patient is unable or even unwilling to speak out. It is the nurse who will have the necessary understanding of what is happening to be able to intervene on behalf of the patient, to express the patient's wishes and defend the patient's concerns if these seem at risk.

In examining the extensive and growing literature which presents the ethics of nursing, there are a number of key questions. The nurse as advocate examines the role of the nurse, especially when the patient is unable or unwilling to have his or her best interests expressed. There is also increasing interest in what is known as *virtue ethics*, which focuses on the question of which virtues are part and parcel of what makes a good nurse. These virtues are not merely professional

---

* Reflecting the variations which different disciplines take in prescribing their approaches to enquiry, this chapter differs from others in its style and omission of the use of references. However, it was felt that it would be useful for readers to be guided to material which may be helpful in their exploration of this subject. Hence the author has provided a suggested reading list which has been included at the end of the chapter.

skills or nursing knowledge but ethical qualities which should be present and functioning in the practice of nursing. At its simplest level this asks what kind of moral characteristics a good nurse should have and how these are to be developed in nursing training and practice.

Recent ethical discussions have inevitably raised difficult questions about relationships with doctors and other health professionals. Matters of confidentiality, where patients have expressed something to a nurse believing that it would go no further and yet the nurse knows that the knowledge may be relevant to the pattern of care indicated by the medical adviser, create problems over what to do with information. Maintaining the confidentiality and trust of the patient may conflict with what may be the patient's long-term interest. Issues of paternalism lie not very far from the surface of such matters.

In practice, nurses are all too often faced with the need to take immediate action, for example in a situation of cardiac arrest, when any decision to resuscitate or not to resuscitate may lead to conflict with the medical staff. Medical staff may well regard such a decision as their prerogative and could disagree with the nurse's assessment of what is best in such conflicts. But the reality is that nurses are often required to make such decisions without being able to refer to medical staff, and this may put them at risk of disciplinary action and even dismissal. Such consequences are themselves part of the moral debate within and concerning nursing ethics, but the moral issues of responsibility and professional judgement for each nurse still remain to be dealt with. Codes of practice and accountability expressed by national nursing bodies usually attempt to deal with these kinds of issues.

Nurses do not make ethical decisions in a vacuum and it is important to understand the wider context in which morality is learned and practised. We shall examine the nature of that context in terms of the knowledge needed, not just for the moral debate but also for ethical decision making.

We all make moral decisions in our work, homes, personal, social, political and professional lives. What is less clear is the basis on which we make such decisions. In this chapter some of the main ethical stances will be explored before comparing the actual differences alternative stances make to professional nursing decisions. The choices we, and other people, make do affect what happens, and much of the difficulty in professional situations arises because of different moral outlooks. It is by clarifying the alternative moral bases and then seeking some way for the resolution of moral conflicts that we can help create harmonious setting and uniform practice.

Principles

For many, morality is a matter of what is obviously right and wrong. Such morality based on principles is called *deontological*. That means we know from the principle what we ought to do. If I hold the principle of the sanctity of life, then I will seek to preserve life in every situation at all costs. Such principle based morality may come from a number of different sources. The nature of the world and human nature may guide us as to what is right and wrong. We know that it is natural to reap what we sow: if I abuse my body with drugs then I must pay the inevitable price. We know that it is good for people if they are touched and that babies and adults respond well to loving touching. It is also unnatural to be alone. We like company and respond to other people. What is 'natural' may guide us in our moral decision making.

Religion is another source of moral principles. Often through some holy book like the Bible, a religion sets out a number of fundamental moral principles to be followed, not only by the adherents of that religious tradition, but by all people. The Ten Commandments are meant for all and contain five fundamental principles which are found in some form or other in every cultural, moral and legal code. The themes covered are:

- Parent–children relationships
- The sanctity of life
- Truth telling
- Sexual ordering in a society
- What belongs to 'me' or 'us' and what does not.

These principles are often held to be self-evident. Anyone who understands what is being suggested will automatically appreciate that these principles are what we ought to do and follow. They are obvious to the morally literate. If we do not understand that it is wrong to kill people just because we feel like it, then there is something seriously the matter with us.

There are two main problems with morality based on principles. The first is where we get such principles from and how we can be sure we have such principles. If I say that I have the right to have a child, where does that right come from? Does it arise because I am a woman and my body is adapted to child-bearing? Does it arise because our society is able to provide me with a test-tube baby if I am having fertility problems or wish to have no sexual relations with a man? Is it a natural right, a societal right, a human right? How would I be able to tell the difference, anyway?

The second problem is how we cope with conflict between principles. If I claim a right to die, can I also claim a right to life? Do I have a right to abortion on demand as well as a right to have a child by any means available? Is a patient's right to choose more important than a nurse's right to refuse to be involved in certain procedures? These conflicts are hard to resolve. A retreat to what is natural is not necessarily helpful. If I believe that homosexuality should be made illegal because it is an unnatural act, there are just as many people who will claim that their homosexuality is perfectly natural to them. How then are we to define what is natural?

Principle based morality is important, but rather than help us solve problems it can create even more.

Consequences

The other main moral theory or set of theories rests on the *consequences* of what we do. What is right or wrong is to be judged by the end-results. If what happens is good, then we ought to do that. If what happens is bad, then we ought not to follow that path. There are two main subsets within this view. They are that each of us should do what gives us pleasure as individuals and that we ought to do what leads to the greatest happiness of the greatest number.

Hedonism

'Eat, drink and be merry for tomorrow we die' sums up the hedonistic outlook. Morality consists in doing what we want. What we want is happiness and pleasure so morality is doing whatever 'turns us on' as individuals. Even the saint and the hero who refuse to behave like the rest of us and resist the cream cakes or suffer for the sake of other people are really doing what they want to do and what gives them pleasure.

The way to make a moral decision is simply to consider what will lead to the happiest consequences for each one of us. It all sounds rather nice and like a good idea. The problem is twofold. There is the joke about the sadist and the masochist: the masochist says to the sadist, 'Beat me! Beat me!' The sadist replys, 'No.' Different people want different things and find different sources of pleasure. How then could we operate a ward, never mind a society, if we all did whatever pleased us? The other problem is that this individualism is the death of a society and of cooperation unless it gives us pleasure. Much of what we do and have to do is not pleasant and we would rather avoid it. It is a nonsense to suggest that I gain pleasure from doing what I have to do.

Utilitarianism

The solution to the selfishness of hedonism is held to be the utilitarian philosophy of Jeremy Bentham and John Stuart Mill. When a Health Authority sits down each year to consider how it will allocate its budget, it may have to decide between spending more money on transplantation units or on care of the elderly. It makes its decision largely on a complex calculation of what will lead to the greatest happiness of the greatest number. Utilitarianism is the idea that what we ought to do is defined by what leads to the greatest happiness of the greatest number. Thus, if giving free syringes to drug addicts leads to more happiness than pain, we ought to do it. If cutting out district nursing services leads to more pain and suffering for more people than the cost benefit gained, then we ought to avoid it.

To follow such a philosophy means that we have to measure pleasure and pain; Bentham designed a pleasure calculus to do that. It measured the duration, intensity, propinquity, extent, certainty, purity and fecundity of the pleasure and pain involved in a course of action. If we end up with more pleasure than pain we ought to follow that course. If the opposite, we ought to avoid it. This moral approach is a practical, down-to-earth means of deciding on social policy, based on seeking the greatest happiness of the greatest number.

There are, however, problems with such an approach. The first is whether or not it is really possible to measure pleasure and pain and whether they are the kinds of things we can add up and take away. Most of us consider that it is more important to alleviate pain than to give everyone a thrill or a bout of pleasure. It is also hard to see how we can add different people's experiences of pain and pleasure together to make some grand total. The situation becomes even more confused if we add Mill's attempt at sophistication by distinguishing quantity and quality of pleasures. Without such a distinction, utilitarianism seems subject to the criticism that it is a 'doctrine fit for pigs'. In other words, the quality of pleasure does not matter. All that is important is getting as much pleasure as possible, so it is better to be a 'pig' satisfied, than Socrates dissatisfied. If utilitarianism does try to distinguish between not just quantity but qualities of pleasure, then it becomes hopelessly complex and arbitrary.

Others suggest that there is much more to morality than pleasure alone. If I close a window in a ward I may please the one sensitive soul who feels the draught and is worried about her rheumatism, but displease the rest of the ward who may not be very aware of draughts but like fresh air. The problem is that we might reach a very different conclusion by measuring the pleasure to be gained by one deeply sensitive soul from the pleasure to be achieved by a large number of less sensitive folk. Should we go for the greatest happiness as defined by the amount, or should we seek the greatest happiness of the larger number even when the actual amount of pleasure may be much less? Either way we end by pleasing the deeply sensitive or doing what everyone else wants, thus becoming the victims of the majority. Mill saw the point and introduced a second theme, that of justice. He argued that everyone should count for one, and no one for more than one. This still leaves us the problem of which principle takes priority in our calculation of consequences, a potential for injustice where the individual suffers for the sake of the majority and a situation where the majority are always right simply by virtue of their numbers.

Consequentialist morality has one further major problem, regardless of whether it is the happiness of the individual or the majority which is at stake. We are not able to predict or control the consequences of our own actions, far less of other people's, so it is hard to see how we can find a solid base for our moral decision making. If morality is nothing more than the results, the decisions we make will be wide open to error as circumstances and consequences change.

It is also widely felt that such a stress on consequences leads to a morality in which the end justifies the means. We can do whatever we like, or feel is justified, as long as it turns out all right in the end. Some would feel that some things are wrong in themselves and ought always to be avoided regardless of the possible good consequences which might (or might not) happen.

Relativism

This is the moral outlook that what is right and wrong varies from time to time, place to place, and person to person. Some primitive societies may eat ageing relatives before they become too frail. This will send them on to the next world able to journey through the land. In British society we put elderly relatives in old folks' homes and visit them occasionally. Morality varies. This implies that there are no absolute standards or rules, but right and wrong are relative to situations and contexts.

Such a society would soon fall apart if everyone did whatever they regarded as right in their own eyes. Thus tolerance is presented as the cure for disintegration. 'Live and let live' should be our motto. You are free to do whatever you wish as long as I am free to do whatever I wish.

At times it does seem as if our society lives by this creed, but it is not without its problems. If I try to argue that everything is relative then am I making an absolute or a relative statement? If it is an absolute statement, i.e. that everything is relative, then it is not true that everything is relative for we have found one absolute statement, i.e. that everything is relative. If on the other hand, it is only relatively true that everything is relative, it is only true for some people at some times in some places and need not be true for me. This is not just a play on words but is showing that there is something fundamentally wrong with the view and the statement of the view, for to try to state it is to fall into a contradiction.

More cogently, such endless variation does not match up with the facts. As we have already seen, there is, in fact, a common core of morality and principles which are universal and basic. Of course, they may well be minimal, but they do offer some objective universal starting point in any moral discussion.

Relativism runs into a further problem in its recommendation of tolerance as a guideline for society, for it moves from describing morality to offering a prescription about how we should live, and that not only requires a new set of arguments, but makes tolerance an universal absolute, thus contradicting relativism itself.

If tolerance is the fundamental virtue, we are in trouble when it comes to dealing with intolerance. How can a society tolerate intolerance, especially if that intolerance threatens the well-being of a society or if it is intolerance of tolerance?

Relativism seems to offer a comfortable moral position but, in fact, does not really help us resolve moral conflicts at all. If there are no absolutes and morality simply varies, then when we try to deal with such variation, relativism offers and can offer no means of resolving that conflict. It merely describes the fact of the conflict without any hope of providing a solution.

Reductionism

There is an unwillingness to face up to the complexity of morality and ethical decision making. Instead, we prefer easy answers even if they are simplistic. The reductionist comes along to help solve our problem. He or she suggests that it is possible to find a simple solution to very complicated problems. Part of the problem, however, is that there are many different kinds of reductionism. Two will indicate the kinds of moves such reductionistic approaches offer.

Marxism

The Marxist suggests that there is one simple way to understand morality and ethical questions. That is to reduce them to economic functioning. Morality is nothing more than a result of economic factors which produce different kinds of morals in different kinds of economic communities and for different roles within an economic community. Clarify the economic issues and you will be able to see the moral issues which rest on those economic factors.

The Freudian approach

The follower of Freud suggests that morality is, in reality, a function of certain basic human needs and desires. Sexuality and aggression are the basic fundamental drives and what we call morality is nothing more or less than ways of coming to terms with these basic urges and needs. Morality will only be successful if it takes proper and full account of such factors and bases itself on those grounds and nothing else.

What such reductionist accounts reveal, and we must remember that there are as many more such approaches as there are philosophies and belief systems, is that behind such views of morality lie very definite accounts of human nature. In essence such accounts are suggesting that the only and complete way to understand human beings is in terms of their particular theory and approach.

Each such view will have problems which are unique to whatever particular account happens to be at issue, but the question for each and every one is to what extent it provides an adequate account of human being. Does it do justice to humanity as we know and experience it? The danger here is twofold. Some reductionist accounts, in their eagerness to carry the day, stretch the facts to fit in with their particular outlook. Others find that all the facts do not quite fit with their framework of thought so they simply ignore the facts which are not so supportive of their view. Either way we need to beware of reductionism which offers apparently simple solutions to complex problems, but in reality is providing simplistic accounts not only of the issue but of the human beings who are at the heart of both the theory and practice of morality.

Individuals, choices and feelings

There are three other moral outlooks which are particularly important in our western liberal society today. They are: existentialism, with its stress on the individual; prescriptivism, with its emphasis on choice; and emotivism, which focuses on the role of feelings in moral decision making.

Existentialism

This is the view that the world in which we live lacks any meaning and purpose. There is no meaning in any one thing and no meaning to be found in everything as a whole. As human beings we are faced with such meaninglessness, often brought home to us in our experiences of suffering and death. Our response may be to try to escape from such reality. We try to retreat into the past and are bound up with the good old days and the way things used to be. Another escape is into the future and we live for tomorrow and look for 'pie in the sky' or in the future there and then. Both escapes are inauthentic to what it means to be a human being. Authentic humanity faces up to the present in the light of the past, but open to the future.

This means that we face up to the lack of meaning and purpose in the world and we create our own meaning. Each of us, as individuals, is responsible for making our own morality. Morality is thus a purely subjective affair. It rests on human choice. It does not matter what we choose, for everything, including our choices, is meaningless. All that does matter is that we choose, and in choosing we commit ourselves 100% with all of our being to living out that choice. Each choice must be made at every moment to be authentic. Our morality is the result of individual choices for we are each to be our own authority and to decide everything for ourselves.

Apart from being a totally exhausting morality, with such pressure on us all to decide all the time, existentialism is flawed in at least two main respects. It isolates us from the community in which we are born, educated, grow up, and live as part of. No one is an island and we live in interdependence with each other. Existentialism also isolates our choosing from the rest of what we are as human beings. Choices do matter. But so also does our thinking and reasoning, our feelings and reactions, our obligations and relationships, which are part of us whether we like it or not and whether we choose them or not. The existentialist account of human nature is too narrow and exclusive.

Prescriptivism

When the Oxford philosophers first read existentialist literature, they were impressed and sure that these Continental philosophers had an important point. The Oxford dons also felt that, like all Continentals, they had exaggerated their case. Thus R.M. Hare produced the philosophy called prescriptivism, which builds on existentialist insights.

Morality is about choices but it is not open to us to choose anything at all, at least in the form of our choosing. Chaos would result. Rather we must all look to Kant's principle of universalizability. When I make a moral choice I must choose what everyone else in the same situation would choose. I cannot beg the question in my own favour. Such choices are essentially rational. In choosing I choose for all men and women. I choose what all reasonable people would choose. In a way, making a moral decision is rather like writing a prescription for what I am to do. When I write the prescription I must write it not just for me but for everybody else who might find themselves in the same situation. This is the way for us all to make our moral decisions.

Hare's account is still subject to some of the problems of the existentialist account, but is also flawed for it seems to separate prescription from description. Not anything and everything can be chosen. There are some things we know to be moral areas and they make demands on us whether we choose to accept those demands or not. It is also hard to see how we can prevent cheating, if I am to choose what everyone else would choose in the same situation. It is all too easy to argue that no two situations are ever the same for no two people are ever quite the same. Thus I can still have one rule for me and one for everyone else.

Emotivism

There is an approach to morality which says that moral decisions have nothing to do with reason or rationality. Morality is about feelings. Thus when I make a moral judgement and call something good or bad I am really telling others what I feel about something. Moral language expresses our emotions and conveys our feelings to people. Some have called this the 'boo–hurray' approach to morality. But emotivism goes a stage further than saying 'boo' or 'hurray'. It also suggests that moral language is used to evoke the same feelings and responses in other people. Thus when I say that 'For nurses to strike is evil', I am telling you how I feel about nurses striking and trying to make you feel the same way too. Thus morality is not about facts but about feelings, and the language we use expresses and evokes emotions.

It is interesting to see how a proper stress can mislead us by trying to make what is a part into the whole. Emotions and feelings are an integral part of morality, for moral issues are things that matter deeply to us and cause strong reactions. But morality is far more than feelings. It deals with facts, principles, consequences, reason and the will, as well as our feelings. Emotivism tells us that morality involves our feelings, but that does not mean that our morality is based solely on these feelings. If it were, and emotivism were true, then any and every means which produced the appropriate feelings would be acceptable and we would be vulnerable to brain-washing and conditioning. These would be acceptable as long as the proper feelings resulted.

A variety of approaches to moral decision making have been critically examined above. It would be wonderful indeed if life were divided up into such neat compartments and people kept in only one such compartment. The reality is that we all tend to move backwards and forwards between these different views without much awareness of so doing or without very much consistency. Yet it is crucial for nurses to recognize these different moral bases and that they, their medical and para-nursing colleagues, their patients and their families and society are all subject to these bases and use them most of the time in making their moral decisions. This will at least give us a means of beginning to discuss and to move to a resolution of disagreement or to create the means of living with that disagreement. But we must try to see what difference different moral outlooks make in some areas of key concern to the nursing profession.

Different moralities at work

Telling the truth

Should a nurse tell a patient the truth about the fact that they are going to die? A principle-based morality might well appear to say 'Yes' for truth-telling is a fundamental rule and principle. This is where such deontological morality reveals its subtlety. The principle might not be simply to tell the truth regardless, but to tell the truth if one is asked. Despite this, it is quite clear that a deontological, principle-based approach to moral issues would lead a person to tell the truth about death and its imminence.

In contrast, a morality based on consequences, especially based on happiness, would tend to ask whether or not a patient would be happier if he or she were to know the situation. On the utilitarian morality, it would not just be the patient's happiness which was involved but those of all involved in the situation. The problem is how we would actually measure such possible happiness. If I tell, then the patient might be glad to know the truth and be able to come to terms with it. On the other hand, the patient might collapse as a result of knowing that death is faced and fall apart. While the consequences obviously depend on how well the nurse knows the patient and the likely response, it is much more complic-ated than that. Doctors may have decided that the patient is not to know, and the consequences of a nurse telling a patient might mean very strained and difficult relationships on the ward for some time to come. The calculation of happiness is not just a short-term business. Nevertheless, it would seem that the consequence-based morality leads to truth-telling only if it will make the patient happy. If telling lies makes the patient happier, then the utilitarian nurse will be free to tell lies to create the greatest happiness of the greatest number.

A relativist and a reductionist would tell the truth or lies according to their particular personal moral view. It might even vary from case to case. This seems like being relevant to individual needs, but masks a lack of the consistency and reliability which are necessary for good nursing practice and the practice of morality.

The existentialist, prescriptivist and emotivisit have no ground rules to draw on here. The existentialist would simply ask for a commitment, so telling lies or the truth does not really matter as long as you choose which one to tell. The prescriptivist does have a rule, which is that everyone in the same circumstances should do the same thing. It is hard to see that we would tell lies or the truth in such settings without thinking that most people would do the same. In the end we tend to be conformist. The emotivist would say it all depends on how we feel. The problem then is that one nurse may feel very differently from another nurse about the issue.

In the end the broad distinction which makes most difference is that between morality based on principles and that based on consequences.

Killing with kindness

The issue of euthanasia is likely to be a growing dilemma for doctors and nurses. Here we are not dealing with all the intricacies of the topic but rather asking whether it is appropriate to allow someone to die by not treating them. It might be an elderly patient with pneumonia or a neonate with severe abnormality and little prospect of an improvement in quality of life.

The deontological approach might hold that the principle of the sanctity of life means that life is to be preserved at all costs. But a different principle might be that of compassion and the relief of suffering. Thus a principle-based morality would lead to different conclusions, depending on the particular principles involved and some hard decisions between competing principles.

A consequentialist approach would ask what will lead to the greatest happiness for the individual and for the community.

This would tend to lead to allowing of someone to die, especially if that could be achieved without pain and distress. Better to die peacefully than to struggle to live painfully.

The relativist and reductionist would tend to support the taking of life, though each might allow keeping people alive if that were part of a subjectively held philosophy and outlook.

The existentialist, prescriptivist and emotivist would tend to concur with the 'allowing to die', though this would depend on the particular outlook again. The prescriptivist might be quite happy to prescribe that everyone in such a situation should be allowed to die. The emotivist would feel that to allow suffering is painful for all concerned and, if we are able to live with the guilt, then the 'allowing of death' is far easier and makes us feel better.

Morality is not a simple affair. There is a wide variety of ethical stances which complicates matters for the nurse trying to understand moral decision making. There may well be crucial differences between personal morality and professional ethics and social and legal standards of what is right and wrong. The nurse will have to come to terms with such differences and decide which have priority over the others. What is crucial in the end is that nurses are aware of the principles at stake, the motives involved (for though the role of motives in morality has not been examined here, it is a key area in making judgements about moral decisions), the nature of the action itself and the likely results and consequences of such actions or failures to act. It is by examining morality in its complexity and in terms of each of these aspects that a nurse is best able to make moral choices and to cope with patients, colleagues and institutions which make different choices.

Further reading

Bandman, E. and Bandman, B. (eds) (1990) *Nursing Ethics Through the Lifespan*, Prentice Hall, New York

Campbell, A.V. (1984) *Moral Dilemmas in Medicine: A Course Book in Ethics for Doctors and Nurses*, 3rd edn, Churchill Livingstone, Edinburgh

Cook, D. (1983) *The Moral Maze*, SPCK, London

Cook, D. (1990) *The Dilemmas of Life*, IVP, London

Davis, A.G. and Aroskar, M.A. (1983) *Ethical Dilemmas and Nursing Practice*, Appleton Century Croft, Norwalk CT

Rumbold, G. (1986) *Ethics in Nursing Practice*, Baillière Tindall, London

Thompson, I.E., Melia, K.M. and Boyd, K.M. (1983) *Nursing Ethics*, Churchill Livingstone, Edinburgh

Tschudin, V. (1986) *Ethics in Nursing: A Caring Relationship*, Heinemann, Oxford

Part Three

Using Knowledge in Practice

The first two sections of this book have concentrated on presenting an insight into some of the sources of knowledge which may be called upon when studying nursing. However, reference has also been made to the special way in which nurses make use of, and often modify, this formal knowledge when in a practice situation. This third section is concerned with sharing some of the experiences of practitioners who have given time and energy to exploring the knowledge base of their practice, teasing out the complex way in which they make use of their knowledge of nursing.

It has been suggested that it is relatively easy to study and learn about nursing or any other practice discipline in the safe environment of an academic institution, but far more complex to make sense of what has been learned when faced with the real world of practice. Indeed Schon (1987) has differentiated between these two settings, describing the former as the 'hard safe ground' where external factors are relatively easily controlled. In contrast, he sees the practice setting as the 'swampy low land' where so many unpredictable and uncontrollable factors impinge on everyday activities that practitioners are continuously having to respond to demands which are unique to a specific situation and time. Consequently they are continuously 'thinking on their feet' and having to find new ways of managing complex clinical problems which do not always fit directly into the theoretical frameworks which have been learned in a more formal setting.

These chapters are concerned with the reality of practice, of making use of 'what is to hand', thus differentiating them from more formal theoretical papers in their eclectic use of knowledge. Indeed, many practitioners are not overtly aware of the vast range of knowledge from which they draw in order to be able to make clinical decisions. This does not mean to say that they do not make very active use of the knowledge which they have gained from theories derived from both nursing and other disciplines. What it does suggest is that very often this formal knowledge is not directly 'applied' but acts as a vital background to help practitioners make sense of the real world in which they work. It also implies that practitioners need to be creative and sure enough in themselves to be able to adjust or modify their understanding of theory, often making use of knowledge in a way which is unique to the particular setting in which it occurs. Sometimes this may lead to the generation of new ideas, when practitioners have the courage to go forward into uncharted waters which have not yet been formally explored.

It is important to emphasize at this point that experienced nurses have always used, and hopefully always will use the knowledge of both their experience and their more formal learning when practising. However, it also has to be said that it is unusual for them to make explicit the sources of knowledge they use in everyday practice. All of the contributors who have prepared the next four chapters have sought ways of sharing their understanding of their own areas of work with the reader. Each one has considerable experience in his or her own field and has explored some ideas in relation to the way in which knowledge has been used.

It has been suggested earlier in this book that it is not possible to express in words everything we know, and this is certainly the case when we are talking about the everyday knowledge of practice. However, through reflection and discourse some of the wealth of understanding can be brought to light and it is with this end in mind that these chapters have been prepared. The authors' ability to pass on all they know is inevitably limited by the written word. However, they do offer some insight into the different ways in which some nurses have sought to make the knowledge base of their practice more explicit.

Reference

Schön, D.A. (1987) *Educating the Reflective Practitioner toward a New Design for Teaching and Learning in the Professions*, Jossey Bass, San Francisco

Chapter 8

Reflecting on care for the mentally ill

Kevin Teasdale

In school, a child will study many areas of knowledge neatly labelled into separate subjects on a timetable. Textbooks present the facts in a clear and authoritative fashion. Frequently, it is only in the years after leaving school that one becomes aware that the neat divisions between knowledge areas cannot be maintained when one is faced with the unpredictable variety of everyday life. The facts are not as clear-cut as they once seemed. Indeed, what were once presented as facts are really only theories, based on more, or sometimes less, evidence.

A similar process of moving from certainty to doubt, and then perhaps to a more limited certainty, is an essential part of becoming an effective member of a practical profession such as psychiatric nursing. With the advent of Project 2000, many institutes are devising new curricula which include all the knowledge areas reviewed in the first part of this book, and more besides. However, a curriculum is an outline document only. The appearance in it of elements of knowledge from many different disciplines conceals incompatibilities between the disciplines in the way in which their theories apply to the mental health field.

For a psychiatric nurse, even the basic question of whether the people being nursed are ill is open to question. Anthony Clare, in his book *Psychiatry in Dissent* (1976), gives two chapters to a review of the controversies between psychiatry, psychology and sociology over the nature of mental health and of mental illness. In summary, some theorists propose that there are distinct psychiatric illnesses with physiological origins which we do not fully understand at present. Others argue that the experiences of the child largely determine the behaviour patterns of the adult. Yet others argue that there is no such thing as mental illness, it is a label used by those with power in society to control others whom they believe threaten their power.

There are also many different therapeutic approaches in use in the mental health field. Each approach is based on assumptions derived from one of these theoretical models. From the illness model follow physical methods of treatment such as medication or electroconvulsive therapy (ECT). Psychological models give rise to talking therapies, of which psychoanalysis is the best known. Some psychologists, drawing on the work of Skinner (1971) and other behaviourists, suggest that it is not necessary to focus on the deeper origins of human problems. It is sufficient to analyse the antecedents and consequences of behaviour, and to modify it using strategies based on rewards and punishments. Meanwhile, sociological studies, such as those of Goffman (1961) on institutionalization, have led to a social policy debate on the influence of the care environment on the mental health of individuals. The argument revolves around the extent to which treatment and care in the safe environment of a psychiatric hospital should give way to community care approaches which keep the individual in touch with everyday living.

How can a psychiatric nurse make sense of such a variety of theories drawn from disciplines with very different basic assumptions and methods of study? Knowledge of what the various disciplines say is not in itself sufficient. The nurse must use personal experience carefully to test the extent to which each theory helps in the understanding of the problems of those being nursed, and to plan effective nursing care. Donald Schon (1983) describes a person who pursues this process of questioning and testing theories as a 'reflective practitioner'.

The core of this chapter is the transcription of an interview with one reflective practitioner. She is the ward sister of a psychiatric day unit, a nurse of fifteen years' experience, ten of those years in different day care settings. In the interview she gives a detailed description of the problems and nursing care of one client, and then reviews her professional practice as a whole, commenting on the place of a day unit in a comprehensive psychiatric service. Each section of the interview ends with a short commentary, highlighting the ways in which the

Ward Sister is drawing on knowledge and experience to plan nursing care.

This account of the client's history has been seen by the client, who has given permission for its publication. Names and some factual details have been altered to preserve the person's anonymity.

Making an assessment

KT (author): Can you tell me how this particular client came to start attending the day unit?

WS (ward sister): Well, the client, Susan, is fifty years old. She is married with three grown-up children. She has never been an in-patient in a psychiatric hospital, and comes to the day unit twice a week at present. Her first contact with the psychiatric services was six months ago. She worked in a large department store on a check-out till. Over a period of months following the death of her mother she found herself becoming more and more vague and unable to concentrate on things. She could feel herself becoming more and more remote from her everyday actions, without being able to do anything about it. It culminated with her being caught taking money out of the till. She knew that the management were watching her, but she wasn't aware that she had actually taken anything. Even at the police station, she was still detached from what was happening, until she looked at herself and realized that to go to work that morning, all she had on was a dress and a petticoat – no tights, no underclothes. 'It was like something clicked, and I realized that I'd snapped. And the enormity of what had happened actually hit me. And I just went hysterical, shouting and screaming I don't know what.' It was this that led her to her GP, and then a psychiatrist being called in to help.

KT: How did you interpret Susan's behaviour, how were you able to make sense of it to yourself?

WS: Even in terms of a reaction to the loss of her mother, it still seemed very difficult to understand. But listening to her talking about her childhood and subsequent events, it began to make more sense. Her mother was the daughter of a fairly wealthy farming family. As a teenager she became pregnant and was forced to marry. The marriage did not work, and she never settled in a permanent relationship. She had a number of illegitimate children by different men, and one of these children was Susan. Her mother sounds like a very cruel person, both physically and emotionally cruel to Susan and the other children. During her childhood Susan suffered beatings, sexual abuse, and overall a lack of love or caring about her feelings. One horrendous example illustrates it all. The family was living in a very out-of-the-way farmhouse. Her mother had a number of miscarriages and stillbirths over the years. The mother used to deal with these herself. One time she had a miscarriage and the baby was obviously dead. Her mother couldn't do anything with the baby until the next day, so she put it in a box and deliberately left it on top of a wardrobe in Susan's room all night.

Susan was about ten at this time. She sat up all night staring at the box, terrified. In the farm kitchen they had one of these large ranges with an open fire. They were way out in the country, and the next morning, to Susan's horror, the mother cremated the baby in the range. This was the sort of terrible thing that Susan grew up with.

Susan somehow managed to survive her childhood, and married young. She seems to have kept the problems and lack of love of her childhood bottled up very much. Some of it did cause problems. It was a long time before the sexual side of her marriage worked, because she felt that if she allowed herself sexual pleasure, she would be becoming promiscuous, just like her mother. The final straw for her was when her mother made advances to her own husband. After this Susan broke off all contact with her mother for many years.

But in old age, her mother reappeared on the scene, and the local council made arrangements for her to be rehoused to be near to Susan. Right up to the end her mother was very cruel to her, sarcastic and interfering. It was then, as the mother was in her old age, that Susan discovered from another relative that the man she had always thought of as her father was not her father! Before she had time to tackle her mother on this, her mother was taken into hospital, and died quickly and unexpectedly. All her life she had played upon her illnesses, and now Susan couldn't believe she was dead. When she saw her there in the hospital bed she cried: 'You're shamming. You can't have left me without answering my questions.'

So you see it was all this family history which had led up to Susan's eventual state. She had kept a huge amount of anger and guilt bottled up all those years. Her mother's sudden death left her feeling alone and in need of help, but with no one to turn to. In this way you can see her taking from the till in the store as a desperate cry for help.

Commentary

This example shows the importance to the ward sister of arriving at an understanding of why the client behaved as she did. She does not resort to an illness model to do this, rather she finds the explanation in what the client tells her about her early childhood. The theories she draws on are those which derive ultimately from a Freudian interpretation of the effects of childhood events continuing into later life. The description of Susan 'bottling up' her emotions is an echo of the Freudian idea of repression. What is unclear at this stage is whether the ward sister rejects an illness model for all her clients, or whether it simply does not correspond with the facts of this particular client's history.

Identifying the problems

KT: Shifting the focus now on to you and the other nurses, how did you decide what sort of care to give Susan? Were you overwhelmed by this history?
WS: Yes, totally. Your jaw just drops open. And really, we looked at her, and you see the family issues, you can't affect in any great way.
KT: What do you mean, the family issues?
WS: Well Susan's three children, she's really gone the other way with. Where her mother rejected and was harsh with her, showing her no affection, Susan's gone the other way. I think to some extent the children, although they are adults now, are still dependent on her for love and approval. Also she has always taken responsibility for their actions, which means they have never really learned to be responsible for themselves.
KT: So how do explain that?
WS: I think that she's giving them all the love that she wanted her mother to give her. She didn't want them to experience what she experienced, so she's gone totally in the other direction. I think she would accept that explanation, without necessarily wishing to do anything really to change it. That's what I mean when I say we must be realistic about what we can achieve here. We do go out to our clients homes now and then, but mostly to make a fuller initial assessment. The work we can do is with the individual client here, but not with the family as a whole because we don't have direct contact with them. The CPNs [community psychiatric nurses] can do work with families, but it's not realistic for us.
KT: So what do you think you can reasonably work on here?
WS: The way we see it, what she wants is the opportunity to sit with somebody, and to be able to talk through and look at her feelings, and examine them, and come to terms with things. And come to terms with her feelings about her mother. I think she's got to the point where she's always kept the lid on it, and she's always been busy with her family and with working to make ends meet. So she's

repressed her thoughts and feelings, particularly about her childhood and her own identity as a separate person ... and then suddenly with her mother's death and her work finished at the store, she had all this in her head. Her husband knew about it, and she used to talk it over with him. But obviously over the years you can't just go on repeating it. So really what we've offered her here is an opportunity to get out of the house a couple of days a week. Out of the environment that's causing her stress. And to be able to ventilate the conflicting feelings she has about her mother.

KT: So the main area you can help her with is to work through her feelings about her mother, and come to see her childhood in perspective?

WS: That's right. And also helping her to find her own identity without always sacrificing her own needs to those of her family.

Commentary

Another major issue in psychiatric nursing appears here: the consideration of who exactly is the client. Should one focus on the individual, or on the family? Starting from work in child psychiatry and psychology, and developing through an understanding of crisis intervention models and systems theory, is the idea that often it is best to regard the family as a single unit. If one tries to help individuals to cope better, it will cause problems or reactions in other family members.

The ward sister is aware of this, and later in the interview gives an example of this happening in Susan's family. However, her concern here is to be realistic. She accepts that in a day care situation she cannot make sufficient contact with the family as a whole to be able to do any useful work. Some of Susan's problems are not amenable to work in this context, even if she wanted to try. This awareness of the limits of effective intervention is the mark of an experienced practitioner exercising professional judgement in the application of knowledge.

The ward sister says that to 'ventilate conflicting feelings' is the key to resolution of Susan's paralysing reaction to the death of her mother. This approach is very much in contrast to the earlier custodial role of the psychiatric nurse, where the emphasis was on managing patients to ensure that emotional outbursts were rare. The theoretical basis for an approach based on ventilation is again linked to Freudian psychotherapy, but further developed in the humanistic tradition of

Carl Rogers (1951), and the co-counselling work of John Heron (1979).

Planning and giving care

KT: Can you tell me now a bit more about what you've actually done to help Susan work on these problems?

WS: It's basically counselling, I suppose. But with minimal intervention. You listen, and really just throw in the odd thing. She's intelligent and she finds her own way. She'll come in one day, and she'll look a bit peaky. And I'll say 'You look a little bit peaky today, do you want a chat? Come on then and we'll go in the group room and sit.'

KT: So you'll do it that way rather than 'I'll see you at two o'clock on such and such a day.'

WS: Yes. We try and do it informally rather than formally. Otherwise it ends up being a bit contrived, and too structured for what she wants. Initially, when she first came, it was virtually, well it was, every time she came – we made time for her. And we sat and gradually, as she's progressed, the amount of time she needs is less and less. We've directed her into things like pottery. And she's discovered that she's quite artistic – things that she never realized. She said 'I never had time for, with the kids ...' and she said that doing things like pottery she's found really beneficial. Because she says: 'If the kids have got me down, and we've had a big family barney, I can really thump the clay, and give it a real good pasting. It gets it out of my system. And it's amazing ... we haven't gone through half so many cups and plates at home! Because I've gone into the kitchen before, and sometimes I get so frustrated at home, I get hold of the door and just bang it, bang it, bang it. It's either that or I fly at somebody, so I do that.' Anyway she goes into pottery, and she's made a magnificent head that she's really proud of.

And she's discovered that she's good at painting and she's been doing fabric painting. She says it gives her release to do things like that. And so we see how she wants to go and then offer her what she feels she needs.

KT: But you offer it, you guide her a little?

WS: Yes, we guide her.

KT: What was your thinking behind pottery or art?

WS: Well, although she does express herself very articulately, I think it's nice to do something creative, and express your feelings in a creative manner. It's just a different way of expressing her feelings and emotions in a more creative way. More positive. She's done all sorts.

She did this magnificent peacock tapestry. She said that she could never ever touch anything like that, because her mother used to do it. And we said, 'Do you fancy having a bash at this peacock we've got?' And she hesitated, 'I don't know'. 'Well we won't push you. It's there if you want it.' And she picked it up and she really got into it. And she said: 'It was like laying a few ghosts to rest.'

KT: Did you know that, when you offered it to her?

WS: Yes.

KT: So it was deliberate?

WS: Yes. To see with things that she had blocks about, to see if she could work it through by doing something.

KT: Have you been doing anything else with her then, apart from the counselling, and the pottery and art work?

WS: We've been doing a bit of assertiveness work with her as well. To sort of, maybe to square her up to the kids. Help her to accept them as mature adults, not as children. They are her children, but they are individual men and women, they're not babies any more. I think that's the hardest thing she's finding at the moment – to accept them.

Commentary

The ward sister briefly, and in a matter of fact way, summarizes a very complex and subtle nursing care programme. One element which emerges is the sense of working with what the client wants and is willing to accept. The use of the word client rather than patient is itself indicative of certain assumptions about the rights of those who attend the day unit. These ideas may be linked to modern social movements concerned with consumer rights. However, in psychiatric nursing they may also draw on the antipsychiatry of Szasz (1974) and Laing (1965). Szasz argued from sociological evidence that our society uses a psychiatric service unjustly, to control individuals whose behaviour we cannot tolerate. Laing worked more from a psychoanalytical tradition, arguing that the words and actions of a person diagnosed as suffering from schizophrenia can be fully understood when interpreted as the continuation of a childhood struggle to establish and maintain a personal identity.

The ward sister is confident in guiding the client into art and pottery. These are not used as occupation alone, but as planned therapy – part of a considered plan to help the client to ventilate her feelings in ways which are constructive. Awareness of the need to pace the client's progress carefully is evident in the gentle approach to offering Susan a chance to work on the tapestry. The idea that it is therapeutic to help a client to express strong, repressed emotions can be found in the humanistic tradition of Heron's (1975) work on catharsis, or the research-based psychology of grief counselling (see for example, Worden, 1983). However, the selection of a tapestry as a creative vehicle for such expression is an example of a nurse using her skills independently and imaginatively, to apply a general theory to the specific problems of an individual client.

One wonders how much of the detail of this therapeutic planning and activity derives from the ward sister's reading, and how much from her experience of psychiatric nursing, and of life in general. Probably she herself is not certain of the balance between the two. What seems to be emerging is a general awareness of progressive themes and recent debates in the mental health field, but not a sterile reliance on academic sources. There has to be an imaginative leap to link theory to the needs of clients. Always the key is the question of whether the approach is 'realistic', whether it produces the desired result.

Evaluating the results

KT: And can you tell me now how Susan is managing and how the care is going?
WS: She's really coming on well. Coming to terms with herself as herself. One thing was when she was going through a really bad patch at home, she had to cover up all the mirrors in her house. Because whenever she looked in a mirror, all she could see was her mother.

But then she came in one day and she was really excited. She threw her arms round me and said, 'I'm so pleased', and I said, 'Go on then, tell us what you're so pleased about', and she said, 'I've managed to uncover the mirror! I went up and I looked at it and said: "You are Susan. You're not your mother. You are your own woman." And I whipped a cover off one, and couldn't look. And then I looked and I saw myself, not my mother. Then I realized that I was almost there.'

And another indication of her progress is that the family are having to adapt.
KT: You mean the family are now having to cope with a different Susan?

WS: Yes. A Susan who is now coming back to as she was, or perhaps a little bit better. Because she's come to terms with a lot of things in her life, and can see things and talk about them. And they find it quite hard to accept and the children particularly are ... 'Oh well mother, it's your illness.' The illness had always been used for the last few months to excuse them from doing what they didn't want to do.

KT: Now, *they* are talking about illness, but do *you* think of Susan as a person who is ill?

WS: No.

KT: How do you think about her? How do you explain her contact with you?

WS: An emotional crisis. I suppose really she was depressed initially. Our first contact with her, she was depressed. Illness? It's always such a statement. I prefer to say to Susan that something's happened in your life, and you're experiencing some sort of emotional trauma. I try not to use the word illness with anybody.

KT: Why not?

WS: Well, it has such ... it's so negative. People then latch on to it, and it's an excuse for everything.

KT: Are there some people here who you think of as ill even if you don't use the word?

WS: Oh yes. Quite seriously ill.

KT: Mentally ill?

WS: Yes, mentally ill. We've got a young man, only 29. He is absolutely heart breaking. This man is a PhD electronics engineer who worked for a computer firm. He is a classic schizophrenic, dreadfully damaged by his illness. He's so damaged that his concentration is a matter of seconds only. He can't sit and read. He's paranoid. He's really ill. Deluded. Very psychotic. And the doctor says: 'There is nothing we can do about him.' I know it's awful to say that at 29 there's no hope for him, but there isn't any hope. He's damaged to such an extent that no drugs, no therapies, no anything will help him.

KT: So what do you try to do?

WS: We just keep him occupied as best we can. When he turns up. And he turns up infrequently. We try and do what we can. I mean, his intelligence is there, but he can't use it because of his illness.

Commentary

In her evaluation of Susan's progress, the ward sister automatically thinks in terms of identifiable behavioural changes.

This is an approach drawn from behavioural psychology, adapted into treatment approaches such as desensitization. But neither the ward sister, nor Susan herself, need to read about the detail of these ideas to understand that uncovering the mirrors is a mark of real progress.

The ward sister elaborates on her view of Susan as not ill but suffering emotional trauma. This is the answer to the earlier question about the extent to which the nurse is relying on a single model to explain her clients' problems. Clearly she is eclectic in her approach. Some of the clients are seen as ill, and a psychiatric diagnosis such as schizophrenia does have value with reference to at least one client. However, although the ward sister uses the illness model to help assess and plan appropriate care for some clients, she does not encourage the clients themselves to adopt this model. She fears that this could make them unnecessarily dependent on medical and nursing services, through seeing themselves as sick or disabled. In this she is clearly drawing on sociological research into role theory, and labelling (see Scheff, 1966, for example).

The ward sister's basis for selecting between models is connected with her view of what can realistically be achieved with individuals. If she, and others, look at clients as ill, their nursing interventions are very limited – given the present state of psychiatric knowledge, with a heavy reliance on pharmaceutical treatments. On the other hand, if some clients are viewed as suffering from problems rooted in childhood traumas, or arising from here-and-now social events within the family, then nursing interventions based on humanistic approaches may be justified. The case cannot be pushed too far however. Some clients are so badly affected that they cannot respond to such approaches. Realistic hope of change is limited with such clients. Thus, although some theoretical models offer greater scope for nursing interventions than others, this ward sister bases her approach on what she sees as the needs of individual clients, rather than on adherence to one favoured theoretical model.

Running a day unit

KT: Now I know that you've worked in different day care settings for a number of years. What views have you formed in this time about the place of a day unit in an overall psychiatric service?

WS: Well, as you know, we have a wide variety of clients here, and they need different things from us.

For example, we do some purely sessional work. We have an anxiety and stress management group for people who come in for that session alone. Really the people we have in that group are what could be referred to as the worried well. They're quite happy to come. And we've managed to get quite a few of them reducing and virtually stopping their minor tranquillizers. And we've encouraged them to form a self-help group outside of here. They telephone each other and support each other. And of course you've got people who've been coming for a while and are now quite well. Who are perhaps just taking two milligrams of diazepam a day instead of fifteen. And they say, 'Oh yes I know just how you feel because six months ago I felt exactly the same. But by doing this, that and the other, and coming here and talking and learning relaxation I have managed to overcome it.' Nothing sells it better. So my role is just as facilitator, helping them to help themselves.

KT: It all sounds very dynamic.

WS: No, I don't think that's quite the right word. Busy perhaps. You see most of our clients don't need anything too intensive. They just need ongoing support. And we've found that, like all day care, you end up silting up with long-term support and maintenance. People who really need minimal nursing intervention, but they do need a social outlet and diversional activities. The trouble is that everybody wants to be a therapist. And what happens to the 60% that need the ongoing support that isn't dynamic? I would love to be a full-time therapist, but unfortunately that isn't going to meet the needs of the majority of my clients.

KT: So what can you do to avoid silting up?

WS: Well I thought that if I didn't do something, we were just going to grind absolutely to a halt. I visited another day unit in a city. They had some good ideas and I could see how they could be made to work better. They had something they called a Link Club, which was really a social club run by the clients themselves. It was a way of weaning them off the main day care, while continuing to meet some of their social needs. So I thought, this is what we need for here. I discussed it with all the clients. And I didn't say to any of them, 'I'm going to cut your days.' I said to them, 'We're going to start this project off. This is what's going to be available – there's going to be chat, and tea and coffee, and games of bingo, beetle drives and stuff. It's going to be on a Monday at such and such a church hall.' We raised money and started a trust fund. Our nursing assistant helps in running it, but the clients themselves have formed a committee and organized things like a trip to the seaside one Sunday. In fact, they're actually coming up to me and saying, 'I know I'm really well now. Would you mind if I don't come to day care any more? If I just go to the club instead?' ... And of course I don't mind at all.

KT: What is it that's made it take off, what is it they see in it that's different from here?

WS: It's not in a hospital. It's theirs. They see it as their club, and it's away from the sick-role environment. Come back here to the hospital, it's the sick-role business rearing its head. That's why I try and not emphasize the sickness aspect.

KT: But here you have a purpose-built day unit in a new general hospital psychiatric unit. Surely it's a superb modern environment?

WS: But wrong for a day unit.

KT: So what's the place for a day unit in a district general hospital like this? Could you close it down and it wouldn't make any difference? Or does it have a value and a place?

WS: My own point of view is that it's totally wrongly positioned. It ought to be in the community. These people live in the community, and to bring them back into a hospital setting is wrong.

KT: But you have to try and make it work?

WS: Yes. But I am lucky. I have some super staff who have stayed with me. And our consultant's great. We've really got a good working relationship. If I make a case for something, he'll listen and respect my judgement. And he talks to me about the referrals first. He'll say, 'I've got somebody I think might be right, what do you think?' and I'll say, 'Well, what are you looking for by sending them?' And then we work it out on that basis. And as part of the care, the medical input is there if we want it, but we hardly ever use it. For most of our clients, a more appropriate approach is, 'Now let's see what you can do for yourself and we can help you.'

KT: Again, that's deliberate? To detach the clients from the medical, illness model?

WS: That's right.

KT: So thinking overall, it sounds as though you get considerable satisfaction from working in day care, despite the limitations of the hospital setting.

WS: I must admit I like day care. I'd be very loath to leave it. I think you've got the best of both worlds really. One foot in the community and one in the hospital.

KT: Thank you very much.

Commentary

In her discussion of the place of a day unit in a psychiatric service, the ward sister shows a detailed understanding of the philosophy of community care which at a policy level derives from the 1975 White Paper, *Better Services for the Mentally Ill* (Department of Health and Social Security, 1975). In fact she goes beyond the White Paper, which advocated day units as part of modern psychiatric units in district general hospitals. Her experience as a practitioner enables her to criticize accepted policy, and in a small way to do something to compensate for its inadequacies.

A strong belief in the importance of self-help comes through also. The emphasis is on the clients' input into the club, as well as the self-support built into the stress and anxiety management group. It is interesting to note that the impetus for the development of the club came from a visit to another day unit. For someone working in a practical profession, being able to see and hear what others are trying to do carries a great deal of weight.

In her relationship with the consultant, the ward sister is a confident professional. She respects his expertise and he respects hers. The day unit, with its particular strengths and limitations, is able to offer a useful service to some clients, but not to others. The ward sister and the consultant negotiate on this as professionals, and agree on the basis of the needs of individual clients. The ward sister has an explicit philosophy of day care. The clients who come are encouraged to see themselves as people with problems, problems which they can tackle if they have appropriate support and are willing to put in some effort themselves.

Conclusion

Researchers in psychology, sociology, or any of the social sciences observe the variety of human activity and construct general theories to explain and predict patterns of behaviour. They work from the specific to the general. A professional in a practical discipline such as psychiatric nursing reverses this process. She studies many general theories, and then tests them out to see whether or not they help to explain the behaviour of individual clients. Whereas the researcher almost inevitably acquires an emotional allegiance to a particular theory, the psychiatric nurse can afford no such allegiance. It does not matter that a theory explains the behaviour of 99% of her clients, if she has the responsibility for planning care for the one in a hundred whom the theory does not fit.

But this does not mean that a psychiatric nurse operates on a purely day to day basis, with no consistency whatsoever. While she must remain open to experience in the explanation of human behaviour, she needs a fixed belief in her own role, and in the therapeutic benefits and limitations of the environment in which she is working. In the case study discussed here, the role of the ward sister is entirely consistent with Virginia Henderson's (1960) definition of the role of the nurse: as a person who helps individuals to become as independent as possible. With an understanding of social policy which enables her to place her day unit in a community context, she is able to encourage clients to move towards self-help, in place of the passive dependence of the sick role. Her task is to create a supportive environment, and to act as counsellor and facilitator. This necessitates forging a link between the generality of theoretical knowledge and the individuality of each client. In this way, a nursing philosophy, and a belief in the therapeutic value of self-help in the community, can be seen to give purposeful direction to the work of one reflective psychiatric nursing practitioner.

Acknowledgements

I would like to thank Gill Wilson, ward sister of the day unit, and Susan, the client. They were both willing to take a risk in talking on the record about themselves and their beliefs.

References

Clare, A. (1976) *Psychiatry in Dissent*, University Press, Cambridge
Department of Health and Social Security (1975) *Better Services for the Mentally Ill*, HMSO, London
Goffman, E. (1961) *Asylums*, Penguin, London
Henderson, V. (1960) *Basic Principles of Nursing Care*, International Council of Nurses, London.
Heron, J. (1975) *Six Category Intervention Analysis*, University of Surrey, Guildford
Heron, J. (1979) *Co-Counselling*, University of Surrey, Guildford
Laing, R.D. (1965) *The Divided Self*, Penguin, London
Rogers, C. (1951) *Client Centred Therapy*, Constable, London
Scheff, T. (1966) *Being Mentally Ill*, Aldine, Chicago
Schon, D. (1983) *The Reflective Practitioner*, Temple Smith, London
Skinner, B.F. (1971) *Beyond Freedom and Dignity*, Penguin, London
Szasz, T. (1974) *The Myth of Mental Illness*, Penguin, London
Worden, W.J. (1983) *Grief Counselling and Grief Therapy*, Tavistock, London

Chapter 9

Caring for the acutely ill

Barbara Vaughan and Mary FitzGerald

This chapter explores some clinical situations where a great depth of knowledge has been used, though not always explicitly recognized, by those concerned. Through reflecting on each of the cases we will try to tease out both the existing knowledge of the practitioners and the areas where they have more to learn. What we hope to be able to make clear is that there is no single overriding source of knowledge which is supreme when dealing with a human situation such as occurs in nursing. Rather that there is both a science and an art in nursing and the skill of practice lies in the acknowledgement and integration of all sources of learning with equal value.

The setting for the first study is an acute medical ward where considerable efforts have been made over the past two years to develop the nursing service, and the majority of the staff have undergone both formal and informal learning during that period of time. They have become acutely aware of the need for enquiry into their practice and the responsibility they carry to continue to learn from their experiences. They are also quite clear about the values they work from and the type of service which they believe they should offer to patients.

In order to explain the context in which the practitioners were working, the first part of this chapter is devoted to sharing some of the background information which explains the way in which the ward functions. The ideas which underlie the practice of the nurses, which they have considered as a team, have helped them to become more critically aware of the knowledge of their practice and gain the ability to examine their work with constructive criticism. The stimulus for changing the way they practise came from many different sources, including the advent of a new curriculum for nurse learners and the appointment of a senior clinical nurse to the unit who was committed to the development of practice and had herself gained considerable knowledge both from experience and from formal learning. Thus leadership came from someone who was aware of the potential service which nurses could offer. With these thoughts in mind, the following section explores some of the underlying issues which made staff on the unit aware of the need to challenge their more traditional ways of doing things and become more conscious of the knowledge base they use in everyday experiences.

Background

Never has the need for nurses to recognize the knowledge base from which they practise been more overt than in recent times. There is a growing pressure for them to become accountable autonomous practitioners (United Kingdom Central Council, 1984; Vaughan, 1989), and whilst this has huge advantages in the degree of interest and motivation it creates for nurses within their work environments, there is also a price which must be paid in terms of the need to expose the rationale for actions.

The pressure which has been put on nurses to change has meant that in many instances they have been asked to move too quickly. Nurses have been used to a traditional model of practice based on rules, policies and tradition, where the origin of decision making was often obscure or delegated upwards to the senior nurse (sister/charge nurse). There have been many instances when decision making was so widely spread that no one nurse could be identified as the person who was responsible, and hence accountable, for an action (Pembrey, 1980). Thus, nurses have frequently been able to avoid exposure of their limited knowledge for prolonged periods of time. Further more, there has been little incentive for nurses to expand their understanding, since their opportunity to exercise discretion in decision making has been severely restricted by the very system in which work has been organized (Pearson, 1988). It is not surprising that, if there is no individual reward, either overtly or through satisfaction in seeing the outcomes of one's own decisions, the drive to develop has been so limited.

It must be remembered, however, that it is not reasonable to expect nurses who have been brought up to work in this traditional way to change overnight and suddenly accept such responsibility. Time is needed to gain both knowledge and confidence (Wright, 1989). Furthermore, it can be argued that expectations arising from such rapid change can be both stressful and highly dangerous. It can also be argued that it is not in the interest of either nurses or patients for nurses to ask for, or be expected to accept, the responsibility of decision making for which they are not prepared (FitzGerald, 1990). However, the counter-argument to this is that nurses do, in many instances, have a huge body of knowledge from which they make judgements; this knowledge has previously gone unrecognized by themselves and others (MacLeod, 1990).

The notion of the autonomous accountable practitioner has been talked about widely in recent time, and on the surface appears very attractive. Despite this wide debate, there is still considerable confusion over exactly what is meant by this term, let alone the implications for practitioners. To clarify this point initially, it is necessary to have a shared understanding of what is meant by such words. First, according to Lewis and Batey (1982), autonomy can be defined as 'the power or right to self govern'. However, they go on to suggest that such freedom only exists *within the boundaries of professional competence*. The implications of such a statement are widespread, for there is a clear indication that autonomy must be limited on an individual basis by the knowledge of each practitioner. Thus, with the advent of a clinical career pattern and primary nursing, we are in a position to acknowledge and reward practitioners as they develop the ability to take on more demanding clinical roles, but also to offer them the opportunity of staying in secure, but therefore less well rewarded posts as assistants to skilled nurses. Johns (1990) argues clearly that these restrictions on autonomy are in fact essential as a safeguard for the consistent and congruent quality of care, and that ways must be sought which limit autonomy without compromising the freedom needed to practise effectively.

Lewis and Batey (1982) also suggest that there is another aspect which relates to the ability of practitioners to exercise discretion in decision making which they refer to as 'attitudinal autonomy', that is when people *believe* themselves to be free to behave in such a way. Thus we can move into the realms of nurses' understanding of themselves, their position within a health care team, their confidence in the soundness of their own judgements and their willingness to live with the uncertainty that sometimes things may not turn out as they had hoped or expected. This is not an attribute which can be gained overnight, nor would such a hasty move be desirable. However, confidence in this area can grow over time and is a prerequisite to expert practice with acknowledgement of the potential contribution of nurses within a multidisciplinary team. While the acquisition of formal theoretical knowledge is one way of supporting such growth there is also a wealth of knowledge which nurses have already acquired and which they demonstrate daily in their practice. Creating an environment which recognizes the value of both formal knowledge and knowledge gained by experience, as well as the limitations of each practitioner and the willingness to be open about acknowledging and repairing knowledge deficits, is an essential starting point for the development of practice itself.

Knowledge in practice

It was with these thoughts in mind that this particular unit began to seek a new way of approaching day to day practice. Raising awareness of the rationale for many of their day to day actions was no easy matter, since in many instances they were unaware themselves of their own ability (MacLeod, 1990). However, they have used *reflection on action* as one means of bringing to the surface the hidden learning which can occur through experience (Schon, 1983, 1987; Boud, Keagh and Walker, 1985; Powell, 1989). Both discussion and keeping journals are common practice amongst the ward staff and are means which they have developed as ways of trying to capture and learn from their own experiences.

It is through reflection on the situation described below that the nurses were able to draw out both their current knowledge and the knowledge deficits which they recognized. As Benner (1984) suggests, the skill of the expert practitioner is in the ability to 'read' the situation and, through a wealth of understanding gained through both formal knowledge and experience, to interpret each unique feature in order to be able to make a judgement. However this 'almost exquisite' sensitivity is not open to analysis in every situation. Indeed, to try to achieve such a level of enquiry all the time in everyday practice would be utterly exhausting and cumbersome and in itself might constrain creativity. In many situations there is little opportunity for reflection at the time because of the speed with which actions occur. However, there is much to be gained by reflection, and this is the opportunity which we have taken here. When someone is new to a situation it is sometimes necessary to compartmentalize things to some extent, which can mean that some of the richness of the whole situation gets lost. Alternatively, as Benner (1984) suggests, in the early stages of learning the whole situation is so complexe that novices cannot make sense of it all at one time, and may lose the very essence of what is happening by not having the background to be able to unravel and make sense of the situation. While each situation is unique, and related to the context in which it takes place, reflecting on that experience can widen the scope of understanding for future action.

The second case study arises from the personal experience of one of the authors. Although the context in which it took place is slightly different, many of the principles which have been described above hold true. Critically, there was a belief in the value of reflection as a means of helping to understand nursing knowledge more fully and a commitment to the development of practice.

Considering practice

As a framework for analysis we have taken the four areas of knowledge described by Carper (see Chapter 1). However, as is often the case in reality, things are not easy to compartment-alize and there is inevitably a degree of overlap. The situations we have used are real (though modified in order to protect the confidentiality of the individuals involved). They act as ex-amples of the manner in which multiple sources of knowledge were used in reality.

Case study: 1

This study presents a complex picture but serves to demon-strate how the depth and breadth of a nurse's knowledge can influence practice. Miss Jacobs was a 79-year-old woman who was admitted to an acute medical ward following a cerebral vascular accident. According to her nephew, up until this time she had led a 'happy and active' life. She was overweight and knew she was hypertensive. On arrival at the ward she was drowsy, with a dense hemiparesis (paralysis down one side), dysphasia (difficulty in speaking) and no gag reflex, leading to an inability to swallow. Miss Jacobs' nephew and his wife came to the ward with her and were obviously concerned about their aunt's condition. Whilst initial attention to Miss Jacobs was appreciated, as the busy evening progressed it was apparent that a tension was growing between the nurses and her relatives. They seemed particularly anxious that any changes in her condition, which they perceived to be an indication of improvement, should be witnessed and acknowledged by the nurses as indicating that there was potential for recovery. They were particularly anxious that she should receive drinks despite frequent explanations about her inability to swallow and the danger of aspiration. Efforts were made to help them to accept this limitation through supporting evidence from medical colleagues who retested her gag reflex during the evening.

Their concern to communicate with their aunt seemed to override all other needs when, for example, having called the nurse's attention to their aunt's wet bed, they continued attempting to talk with the nurse for a further twenty minutes whilst she waited to attend to the patient. The nurse understood the importance of their needs and was anxious to allow them space to talk during this time, despite the business of the ward, but could feel a personal tension rising that was becoming increasingly difficult to manage.

Over a period of time, as the nurse's *understanding* of the situation developed, it appeared to her that the relatives' greatest fear was that active intervention was going to be stopped. It appeared, by their behaviour, that they felt signs of recovery, which were not obviously apparent, would be missed and there was a lack of trust that action would be taken, not only to see to Miss Jacobs' comfort but to preserve her life. In time they made it clear that despite the severity of their aunt's condition and the limited potential for her recovery they would not give up hope and were seeking evidence of active intervention from all members of the health care team.

This view was not necessarily at one with that of the clinical staff, who felt that there are times when people have the right to die with dignity without being subjected to potentially degrading, life-prolonging measures. Furthermore, they were, aware that there was little that could be done to improve Miss Jacobs' clinical condition.

Analysis

The situation which had arisen was obviously complex, creating tension and anxiety on both sides. However, one way of helping the nurses concerned to come to terms with what was happening was through an exploration of the knowledge they were drawing on in order to decide how best to nurse the family. Using Carper's four patterns of knowing, we can begin to unravel some of their thought processes.

Empirics. An understanding of the physiological and pathological changes which had occurred gave insight into Miss Jacobs' prognosis. She suffered from hypertension and was overweight, which suggested that she was likely to have disseminated vascular disease. Furthermore, she was at above average risk of developing the complications of immobility resulting from her stroke, such as chest infection, urinary stasis and thrombosis. These gave potential for both short-term and long-term difficulties in the process of rehabilitation. However, what was of greater immediate concern was the extent, nature and postion of her cerebral infarction. Not only was she at high risk of a further bleed or extension of the current infarction but there is evidence to indicate that the likelihood of the recovery from a stroke of this nature is poor (Weatherall, Ledingham and Warrell, 1987). From this knowledge the nurses were able to understand that the limits of our technical ability are such that nothing could be done to improve her physiological prognosis.

Art. If a purely physiological stance had been taken the nurses would have been able to provide a service that did nothing more than keep Miss Jacobs comfortable, clean and hydrated, and the problem would have been resolved with a clear conscience. However, from their perspective of what nursing is, influenced to some extent by their understanding of the sociological theory of families, they did not see Miss Jacobs as their sole client and felt that they had a responsibility to offer a service to the family as well. The difficulty arose in the apparent tension which was developing between the family and the nurses, despite every effort being made to provide support, comfort and understanding through what was evidently a difficult time.

An important observation from this situation was the clarity with which this group of nurses understood the extent of their role. They were quite united as a group in seeing that they had a direct responsibility to try to help not only Miss Jacobs, but also her family, demonstrating their shared understanding about what nursing 'is'. They were confident in defining their responsibility as nurses and clear that nursing is concerned not only with the patient but also with the family unit (Orem, 1985).

It was at this stage that empirical evidence from a different source was drawn upon. First their knowledge of the psychological theories of grief and loss helped them to understand some of the relatives' behaviours. However, apparently intuitively, this seemed insufficient to give a total explanation of the situation and returning to the information available led them to begin to query whether there were some sociocultural issues which might help them to understand what was happening and therefore offer a more sensitive service.

Miss Jacobs and her family were Jewish. While none of the nurses had a full understanding of the cultural norm within the Jewish community, they were aware that views regarding the sanctity of life are strong. They began to suspect that the notions of quality of life were tempered by a belief in survival at all costs. While at this point in time they were not able to verify their interpretation, it gave them a working framework to gain insight and plan the skilful intervention necessary to help this family. Spicker and Gadow (1980) talk of the nurse's role as advocate for a patient when the nurse helps a patient to voice his or her views. However, they acknowledge that this is most difficult when the patient is silent, and criticizes the tendency to beneficence (acting in a way you think is in the patient's best interest) on these occasions. The nurses genuinely believed that in this instance the family were more likely to be able to know what their aunt would wish even though they found it uncomfortable. Because of this insight, the care which they offered this particular family had to be modified and, despite a superficial likeness of this family situation to many other cases, it became apparent that a different intervention was required.

Personal. Asking people to behave in a way that is contrary to their personal beliefs and values will inevitably create tension. However, drawing on the work of such people as Rogers (1983) and Peplau (1952), the nurses had, over a period of time, come to understand how important it is to respect and understand the client's perspective. By acknowledging their own feelings, beliefs and values in this particular instance they were able to understand the tension that had arisen and, through this understanding, collectively respect the family's view but still live comfortably with themselves. Sharing their experiences and thoughts with one another dispelled the feelings of anxiety and failure which can arise so easily in a situation of this kind and helped them to gain a greater insight which they will hopefully be able to use in their future practice.

Moral. It can be argued that morality is a vague and ill-defined subject which may be based on both rights and duties. In this instance, the nurses perceived that the very nature of their duty was to give respect to the individual patient and the family's rights. However, in this particular situation this did not mean that false hopes were raised by giving unrealistic reassurance that would have denied their understanding, through empirics, of the physical situation. What it did mean is that they could draw on knowledge from the behavioural sciences to plan the service which they offered, taking into account the feelings of loss and fear which frequently arise in a situation of this kind to help them to understand the family's needs. While sanctity of life is true to most cultures, the way in which this is interpreted can vary. Recognition that there is no right or wrong answer to many moral dilemmas can go some way to helping people to gain respect for one another, even when their views differ.

An important consequence of this situation was acknowledgement on the part of the staff of a deficit in the knowledge they required in order to be able to offer full and well-balanced nursing care. As an outcome, literature was sought to deepen their insight into the many religious and cultural variations which are reflected in their local population. Lessons were learnt about the benefits of reflection which, on this particular occasion, was used as a problem solving mechanism. Giving acknowledgement to the presence of tension and reflection on the possible causes enabled them to prevent what could have been an unhappy and damaging situation from arising.

(Miss Jacobs died a few days later, quietly and peacefully. Her family had spent a considerable amount of time not only with her but also with the nurses. A mutual trust and respect grew over this period, so that support could be offered through a deeper understanding of individual needs.)

Case study: 2

This case study presents what appears at first sight to be a very straightforward situation concerned with assisting a patient in taking her prescribed medication. Mrs Edwards was a lady in her middle fifties who had prided herself all her life on 'not needing to go to the doctor', having enjoyed good health. Over the years she had come to learn to manage her own minor symptoms well and developed many 'home remedies' for the various aches and pains which everyone suffers from time to time. She had also developed an acute dislike of taking any form of pill or potion which she saw as potentially harmful, preferring to resort to relaxation rather than paracetemol when she had a headache.

Now she was faced with a dilemma. She had been diagnosed as having a form of diabetes which required daily insulin injections and the responsibility for teaching her how to administer her own insulin lay with the nurse. At first sight Mrs Edwards' problem would seem straightforward; that is, learning to administer the injection and readjust her life-style to accommodate to her newly diagnosed diabetes. However, some knowledge (limited here by an understanding that not all knowing can be expressed in the written word) of Mrs Edwards' background suggested that there was much more than a physiological and technical need in this situation.

The question raised was the extent of the nurse's responsibility in this situation. It could be seen as ending once Mrs Edwards had learned to administer her injection competently and learned about such things as dietary control and exercise in relationship to her diabetes. However, the broader view of nursing taken in this unit led the nurse caring for her to be concerned about the way in which this diagnosis might be perceived and understood by Mrs Edwards. Thus a different picture emerged which called on a much broader range of knowledge. The nurse's *personal* understanding of her role and responsibility in this situation influenced the way in which she worked. However, it must be added that her understanding of this role was not dependent solely on her personal view but had also been influenced by the knowledge she had gained through learning about how others see nursing. Thus an element of tenacity, authority and a priori knowledge (see Chapter 1) had all come into play in her current understanding of her role.

Moving on to this specific situation, it is possible to see how a vast array of knowledge was needed to help Mrs Edwards. There was the *empirical* knowledge, of diabetes itself and the range of factors which would influence her physiological well-being. In the same way the nurse drew on her knowledge of how people learn, taking into account both teaching and learning theory but also drawing on her range of clinical experience in 'getting the timing right' (Benner, 1984) and judging when and how Mrs Edwards would be most open to learning (*artistry in practice*). Whereas previously she might have been satisfied with a 'standard' teaching programme, she sensed that the difficulty for Mrs Edwards was not in learning the skills required to monitor and control her diabetes, nor in understanding the complex clinical management of her new condition, but in coming to terms with the fact that she would be dependent on taking insulin for the rest of her life. She would have to make major adjustments, not just in her life-style but also in the way she viewed life: an aspect of *personal knowledge* for both Mrs Edwards and the nurse.

Opening up the chance to talk brought to light the dramatic effect that this new diagnosis had had on Mrs Edwards' value systems. Her previous image of herself was centred on someone who was fit, healthy and quite able to manage her own health. She perceived that she had done everything she could to maintain this situation. Yet here she was with a 'chronic disability' (her words), which was not only beyond her control but would also make her dependent on others. Thus she was experiencing guilt and anger as well as anxiety about her situation. Drawing on her understanding of loss and bereavement, the nurse began to gain a greater insight into Mrs Edwards' needs. This led her to adjust her intentions in order to try to address some of these issues. Her actions were already planned to maximize Mrs Edwards' ability to care for herself but she also recognized that she might need a deeper understanding of the physiological condition than some people require in order to return a feeling of self-control. Similarly, explanations of the aetiology of the disorder might help in reducing the self-blame.

More importantly, she felt that it was important to work on the notion of dispelling the myth of 'chronic disability'. It would have been easy to offer platitudes of either sympathy or dismissal of the perception as being unrealistic: what Peplau (1969) calls 'pseudo closeness'. However, in this instance the question it raised for the nurse was how she viewed people who had to face this difficulty. Did she see them as 'disabled', and if this was the case would she subtly reinforce Mrs Edwards' concern? This led her to reflect on what her personal feelings would be in Mrs Edwards' situation and to raise questions with her colleagues as to how both they and she viewed people who were dependent on taking medication for their well-being. Such questions as whether they are 'well' or 'ill' were raised. Are they able to lead a free and independent life and could they, for example, take on jobs such as nursing, with its erratic hours and fluctuating physical demands? As is often the way in such circumstances, the personal experience of a colleague was able to help this nurse to develop her own understanding. It came to light that a colleague shared a flat with someone with diabetes, a young healthy adult who lived a full and busy life. With Mrs Edwards' agreement, arrangements were made for her to visit the ward and share some of her experiences, not just with Mrs Edwards but also with the nurse. Thus her acknowledgement of a gap in her *personal* knowledge, even though she knew the *empirical* knowledge related to diabetes well, led her to take actions to try to deepen her understanding of how she perceived this difficulty.

(When Mrs Edwards left the ward she was well able to handle the physical aspects of her diabetes but, more importantly, was openly prepared to face this new challenge in her life. Obviously time was still needed for her to establish a 'new order of things' but many of her fears seemed to have been dissipated and some of her old determination and optimism was evident.)

Epilogue

These case studies only begin to explore the depth of knowledge which was both used and gained by the nurses who were involved in the situations outlined above. As Polyani (1958) says, we can never tell all that we know. Even now, as we reflect on these particular stories, we gain further insight into the complex world of nursing work. In the same way, new insights which were not apparent to us or included in the description may have become evident to you as you learned something of our experiences. Unfortunately it is not possible for us to share all of our learning with you, the reader, since you did not actually live through the experiences with us. The proposition knowledge which becomes available through the written word can only touch the surface of the learning which occurred. The 'tacit' or hidden knowledge which leads to personal growth and development of those who have actually experienced a situation is something that cannot always be made explicit but should never be underestimated. There is no way in which others can either teach or demonstrate overtly all that they know. To benefit by such learning each practitioner must actively engage in the critical enquiry of his or her *own* experience, as did the practitioners involved in these studies.

Nevertheless, we hope that we have been able to present sufficient evidence to demonstrate the value of reflection on action as a means of enhancing nursing knowledge. Our experience suggests to us that this type of learning is one way of making theory come alive. It is so easy to lose sight of the meaning of theory when immersed in practice, or alternatively to become constrained by rigid adherence to textbook theory. Through reflection, there is a shift from the mere 'application' of theory to the 'use' of theory: that is, making it work for you as a backdrop to the decisions that are made in the real world of nursing. Through means such as this it may be that new nursing knowledge could emerge for the future.

References

Benner, P. (1984) *From Novice to Expert* Addison-Wesley, Menlo Park CA

Boud, D., Keogh, R. and Walker, D. (1985) *Reflection; Turning Experience into Learning*, Kogan Page, London

FitzGerald, M. (1990) Autonomy for practicing nurses. *Surgical Nurse*, **36**, 24–26

Johns, C. (1990) Autonomy of primary nurses: the need to both facilitate and limit autonomy in practice. *Journal of Advanced Nursing*, **15**, 886–894

Lewis, F. M. and Batey, M. V. (1982) Clarifying autonomy and accountability. *Journal of Nursing Administration*, **12(9)**, 13–18

MacLeod, M. (1990) Experience in everyday nursing practice. PhD Thesis, Edinburgh University

Orem, D. (1985) *Nursing Concepts of Practice*, McGraw Hill, New York

Pearson, A. (1988) *Primary Nursing — Nursing in the Burford and Oxford Nursing Development Units*, Croom Helm, London

Pembrey, S. (1980) *The Ward Sister — Key to Nursing: A Study of the Organization of Individualised Nursing*, Royal College of Nursing, London

Peplau, H. (1952) *Interpersonal Relations in Nursing*, G. P. Putman, New York

Peplau, H. (1969) Professional closeness. *Nursing Forum* **8(4)**, 342–360

Polyani, M. (1958) *Personal Knowledge*, University Press, Chicago

Powell, J. (1989) The reflective practitioner in nursing. *Journal of Advanced Nursing*, **14**, 824–832

Rogers, C. (1983) *Freedom to Learn for the Eighties*, Merrill, Columbus OH

Schon, D. (1983) *The Reflective Practitioner*, Basic Books, New York

Schon, D. (1987) *Educating the Reflective Practitioner*, Jossey-Bass, Oxford

Spicker, S. S. and Gadow, S. (eds) (1980) *Nursing; Images and Ideals — Opening Dialogue with the Humanities*, Springer, New York

United Kingdom Central Council for Nursing, Midwifery and Health Visiting (1984) *Code of Professional Conduct*, UKCC, London

Vaughan, B. (1989) Accountability and autonomy. *Nursing Times*, **85(3)**, 54–55

Weatherall, D. J., Ledingham, J. G. and Warrell, D. A. (1987) *Oxford Textbook of Medicine*, vol. 2, University Press, Oxford

Wright, S. (1989) *Changing Nursing Practice*, Edward Arnold, London

Chapter 10
Developing clinical standards

Christopher Johns

Every day in clinical practice nurses use knowledge to guide the actions they take, although very often they are not consciously aware of it. However, Clarke, (1986) has defined a nursing action as 'an action deliberately thought out for the benefit of the patient'. If we accept Clarke's definition, then it follows that nurses should consciously make decisions about their actions and, in doing so, make choices from alternative possibilities which are created from various sources of knowledge. One way of identifying these sources and making them explicit is through the process of developing *standards of care* which can be defined as: 'A professionally agreed level of performance suited to local practice that is both achievable and desirable, and able to be monitored' (adapted from Kitson, 1986).

The process of developing standards is fundamentally a problem solving exercise (Kitson, 1989) which involves nurses in reflecting on, and challenging, their existing practice and the knowledge base upon which it is founded. This scrutiny of the rationale for practice can, in turn, lead to a seeking out of relevant knowledge-based criteria, which can be categorized in three groups: structure, process or outcome criteria (Donabedian, 1968).

Structure criteria describe situations that are considered necessary prerequisites to enable an agreed level of performance to be achieved. *Process* criteria are generally actions that need to be made by health workers to achieve that level of performance. *Outcome* criteria are indicators that a level of performance has or has not been achieved (Kitson, 1986). They may be described in terms of various behaviours or levels of satisfaction by patients or their carers, or else in terms of organizational and professional issues. These three groups of criteria are, of course, interdependent.

This chapter will illustrate how the knowledge base of practice can be explored through developing a standard of care concerned with respite care. From this specific example, readers should be able to identify various sources of knowledge that are relevant in all practice situations, although in the example given the *mix* of knowledge is specific to the local setting. The different sources of knowledge which may be drawn on in this instance are concerned with:

- Knowledge of disease and associated anatomy and physiology which may effect either the patient or carer.
- Knowledge related to the demands of the local community on the hospital's resources. For respite care this includes knowing the extent to which dependent people are cared for by carers within the local population served by the hospital, and encompasses the information of epidemiology and morbidity.
- Knowledge of the meaning of illness and the stress of caring, for the patient and the carer.
- Knowledge of person, including social and psychological factors that are significant in understanding people as members of a social and cultural community.
- Knowledge of the values, beliefs and attitudes of nurses and other appropriate health care personnel such as social services workers and doctors who work with dependent people and their carers.
- Knowledge concerned with issues such as the rights of patients, and wider social welfare issues, including access to support services and hospital admission.
- Knowledge of available resources which are required to enable the needs of patients and carers to be planned and met. This includes the repertoire of interventions the nurse can choose from and use with patients, as well as structural issues in providing a service, such as the number of beds available, budget constraints, and the establishment of nurses. Structural knowledge of this nature is influential in determining whether desired standards of care can be achieved.
- Knowledge of self which guides motivation to act, confidence to act, capability of acting, and actual behaviour, where the effect of the self on others is known to be

associated with personal feelings. This knowledge is largely drawn from psychology but may also include an understanding of the social knowledge of organizations, which may help in exploring the relationships between different health workers.

- Knowledge of research or evaluation which has demonstrated effective strategies for recognizing and meeting the needs of dependent people and their carers.
- Knowledge which enables the nurse to choose appropriate interventions. This knowledge is developed through logic, sensed intuitively, gained through experience, particularly of similar events experienced previously, and influenced by education and socialization. These factors can be described collectively as professional judgement. The knowledge also encompasses skilled performance, that is knowledge of personal performance, both of a technical nature concerned with specific tasks and of an interpersonal nature concerned with developing relationships with others. Benner (1984) describes clearly how nurses operate at different levels of competence depending on knowledge of personal performance to guide action and their choice of interventions.

From the personal experience of supervising primary nurses at a small community hospital, it would seem that nurses have a tendency to make interventions based on three groups of criteria:

- Those they already know
- Those they know have worked before
- Those they are comfortable in using.

These criteria may, however, be inappropriate within Clarke's definition of a nursing action, which calls for critical reasoning.

Knowledge and standards

All these sources of knowledge can become combined in a sensitive way to produce a practice situation which is reflected in a standard of care statement. The standard of care (Figure 10.1) described here was developed at Brackley Cottage Hospital as part of the strategy employed to turn the hospital's philosophy for practice into reality. Two key elements of this philosophy are:

- Understanding the role of the cottage hospital in meeting the health care needs of the local community.

All carers of dependent people (who are suitable for hospital admission) are able to arrange respite care with the hospital for a maximum of two weeks at any one time

1.0   Structure criteria

.1   Two beds set aside for respite care

.2   Diary system for 'booking' patients

.3   GPs accept that any carer can refer to the hospital although initial acceptance has GP approval

.4   Hospital's operational policy reflects this usage of beds

.5   Criteria for what constitutes 'suitable for hospital admission':
(a)   Has Brackley GP (unless cover arranged through a Brackley GP)
(b)   ? Only one patient with KTC score < 18 at one time
(c)   Does not exhibit overt antisocial behaviour (at senior nurse's discretion)

.6   Information booklet available

.7   Developed respite care assessment form that recognizes both the patient's life-style and the carer's needs.

.8   Nursing knowledge of carer needs (resource file)

.9   Patient always assigned to the same primary nurse

2.0   Process criteria

.1   Nurse will check availability of bed and book patient on to diary

.2   Patient's GP informed (if referral not through GP) of need for hospital admission

.3   Primary nurse will visit patient and carer at home (if considered appropriate) prior to first respite care admission

.4   Respite care assessment form sent to carer prior to admission

.5   Primary nurse will use the assessment form as basis for discussion of care with carer, to plan and give care

.6   Primary nurse will assess how the carer is coping to identify need

3.0 Outcome criteria

.1   Carer obtains relief of care

.2   Patient's normal life-style is minimally disrupted

.3   The carer is confident about the relative coming into hospital

.4   The carer has coping resources identified and met to enable more effective coping at home

.5   The carer's role as prime carer is recognized by feeling involved in the care process

.6   The carer indicates satisfaction with care

Figure 10.1   Example of a standard of care statement: respite care access

- Defining the meaning of nursing for nurses who work together at Brackley Hospital.

This 'meaning of nursing' is again sensitive to the local situation, although influenced by the current ideology in nursing and the various sources of knowledge that impinge on this ideology.

The influence of the nurses' definition of nursing at Brackley is not overtly recognized within the criteria of this standard, although the role of the hospital in meeting the need for respite care can be recognized clearly. Because standards of care are directly related to the philosophy for practice, the influence of the way in which the nursing staff defined nursing has been assumed.

Details of each of the structure criteria are given below in order to demonstrate the way in which they were developed. Less detail has been included about process and outcome criteria as the same principles were adhered to as they were prepared.

Structure criteria

1.1 Two beds set aside for respite care

The hospital has 13 beds and serves eight general practitioners (GPs) for a fast-growing town and surrounding villages. Of the 350 cottage or community hospitals in England and Wales, 86% provide a respite care service (Tucker, 1987). The government has recognized the significance of this type of hospital in providing respite care (Department of Health and Social Security, 1975). Considerable evidence exists that carers lack support, both in terms of services within their homes and in getting relief from care.

A retrospective 6-month analysis of the use of the hospital's beds for respite care patients was undertaken at Brackley and indicated an average occupancy of 1.2. Over this period the service had been arranged on an *ad hoc* basis in response to requests from the general practitioners. It was assumed a greater demand could be generated by both encouraging more potential carers to use the service, particularly through direct referral to the nursing staff, and by arranging respite care on a regular basis, i.e. one week in every six weeks. Based on this assumption, it was was decided to set aside two beds for respite care. No demographic study was undertaken as no indication of recommended respite care beds per unit of population was found. Analysis over the six months following the writing of this standard demonstrated an increase of occupancy to 1.8 patients, i.e. 90% occupancy, justifying the allocation of two beds. Occupancy of the total hospital beds fluctuated between 70 and 100%, indicating that other demands would make it difficult to offer more than the two beds for respite care even if demand indicated this. This analysis of bed usage illustrates one way in which empirical knowledge can be generated. The need for respite care had also to be weighed against other needs for other categories of patients for whom the hospital provided a service.

1.2 Diary system for 'booking' patients

The use of a diary system enabled the nurse accepting a booking to see when a bed was available. The hospital had a tradition of responding to demand from carers which the staff wanted to maintain. Two other respite care schemes in local hospitals were examined and compared with two descriptions of schemes from the literature. In all four schemes care was organized between set days, and in two schemes only on a planned basis for a set number of families. The advantage of these systems was a 100% bed occupancy but at the disadvantage of flexibility and response to carer need. However, these issues were seen as crucial to the service and a policy of responding to carer need, whilst encouraging regular relief, was agreed by the nursing staff as preferable. To make this decision effectively it was crucial to obtain feedback from the carers themselves as to their needs. The decision could then be based on knowledge from carers rather than from assumptions about what carers might want. By obtaining this feedback it is possible to begin to explore the tension between nurses prescribing what they consider is beneficial to patients and carers, as opposed to what patients and carers may identify for themselves.

1.3 GPs accept that any carer can refer to the hospital, although initial acceptance has GP approval.

This criterion necessitated a negotiated agreement with the general practitioners that nurses could control admission and discharge for this group of patients. This enabled the primary nurses to plan relief of care with relatives with the knowledge that they had freedom to practice, limited only by the structural constraints imposed by the diary. The negotiation demonstrated a traditional power relationship between the general practitioners and the nursing staff, where the general practitioners controlled all aspects of admission and discharge of patients. However, empirical knowledge of carer need proved compelling in changing this power relationship. This knowledge can be described as tested knowledge.

This example illustrates how developing such knowledge supports assumptions made about providing a service and the nature of caring. The knowledge was also significant in changing the structural and attitudinal autonomy of the nursing staff, enabling them to change the traditional power relationships with the general practitioners. Knowledge from medical sociology suggests that this is a difficult thing for nurses to achieve. Webster (1985), for example, found in his study of medical students that the vast majority seemed to assume that nursing is essentially a lower level of the practice of medicine, entirely dependent on the physician's instigations. Knowledge of medical sociology also reveals a consistent story of the professional dominance of medicine over nursing and other health professions (Friedson, 1970). Furthermore, social research has suggested that nurses are powerless to change this status quo, socialized as they are into subordinate roles (Buckenham and McGrath, 1983).

The psychology of communication between nurses and doctors can also contribute to understanding. For example, work undertaken by Stein (1978) illustrates how doctors and nurses play communication games that reinforce the role of the doctor as decision maker.

To set criteria within a standard that explicitly challenges the control of medicine in making decisions can only be achievable within the security that knowledge brings. In this respect, knowledge is power. Although this particular knowledge is not directly related to the practice situation of caring for respite patients and their carers, it does illustrate the background knowledge necessary to consider whether a standard is achievable or not. These factors can be described as the extrinsic environment of care in relation to developing a philosophy for practice.

1.4 Hospital's operational policy reflects this usage of beds

Writing a policy for respite bed usage confirms verbal agreements made amongst staff and enables them to proceed confidently and consistently 'within the knowledge' that this has been agreed.

1.5 Criteria for what constitutes 'suitable for hospital admission'

(a) Has Brackley GP (unless cover arranged through Brackley GP)
This criterion again demonstrated the need for a multidisciplinary approach to writing standards of care. Where 'vacancies' were demonstrated on the respite care diary, the hospital could accept referrals for patients with a non-Brackley GP, provided that the patient's own GP had arranged local cover.

(b) Only one patient with KTC score < 18 at one time
The hospital did not use a dependency tool to measure the nursing workload. Staff intuitively knew what they could manage. However, being nurses, they had always 'coped' and taken much satisfaction in this, despite protestations at times when 'things were heavy'. Workload should be an important consideration in accepting patients for respite care. Much evidence exists, particularly in relation to residential homes, that populations are becoming more dependent. This is probably also true for community hospitals. Empirical knowledge that gives weight to this assumption within community hospitals is based on interview data (Johns, 1989) but where no evidence exists to support assumptions, it may be incumbent on nurse practitioners to justify decisions through collecting information of this kind. Knowledge derived from this information is not usually widely applicable but does provide valid insight into the local practice situation.

Analysis of dependency using the KTC formula (MacGuire and Newberry, 1984) indicated an average dependency level for this group of patients only slightly higher than the average for other patient groups. However, the criterion reflects a concern to avoid the admission of two high dependency patients at one time (< 18 score) due to workload considerations. The 'spin off' from using this tool may be to confirm staff intuition of 'heaviness' and to use findings to argue for increased resources where necessary. Managers are more likely to listen to 'hard facts' than nursing intuition. This last comment is also written intuitively!

(c) Does not exhibit overt antisocial behaviour (at senior nurse's discretion)
Admission of some patients suffering from dementia was considered inappropriate because of their potential effect on

other patients through 'antisocial' behaviour, or because of the attention they required, particularly those who wandered. The problem was compounded by lack of knowledge and skill in caring for patients with this kind of problem, tinged with the expression of some difficulty in caring for confused people. However, the nurses found it impossible to set criteria against which to judge 'antisocial' behaviour: each patient had to be assessed on personal merits. New referrals with this kind of problem can be visited in their homes for assessment, but most of those referred are accepted despite probable difficulties, and a decision made subsequently, in the light of review, as to suitability for further admission. A major ethical problem for the staff is that carers of this type of patient are often most in need of a break. In some cases a compromise is agreed, restricting the stay to one week.

Discussing the practice situation of respite care did highlight both restrictive attitudes by staff and lack of knowledge in caring for confused patients. Access to research was helpful in relation to attitudes. A teaching session was arranged about 'unpopular patients', with particular reference to Stockwell's research (1972). This work illustrated how nurses reject and accept patients from an applied psychological perspective. It raises potentially important issues for the assignment of primary nurses to patients and of nurses being aware of their feelings about patients. Many patients accepted for respite care are very dependent and fit Stockwell's description of unpopular patients well. More recent local work has also indicated that patients who are unable to engage in meaningful conversations with nurses may be labelled unpopular with staff (Johns, 1989). This is, however, an example of research undertaken within one location and the extrapolation of the findings to other nursing areas cannot be assumed.

The issue of nurses feeling capable of caring for respite care patients and their relatives may seem trite, but self-awareness is crucial for nurses in providing therapeutic care for this or any other group of patients. Psychological knowledge demonstrates (Menzies, 1960; Jourard, 1971) that nurses take active measures to protect themselves from the anxiety of working closely with patients; this does little to encourage working therapeutically or, as Clarke (1986) says, 'for the benefit of the patient'. Bergman (1981) believes that nurses should only accept responsibility for work they have the knowledge and skills to cope with, otherwise it leaves them vulnerable in being held accountable for their actions. Such a view is just as pertinent when considering relationships as in any other aspect of care.

1.6 Information booklet available

An information booklet was written to give both patients and relatives information about the hospital. Recall of verbal information, particularly when the recipient is anxious, has been demonstrated to be poor (Lane-Franklyn, 1974).

1.7 Developed respite care assessment form that recognizes both the patient's life-style and the carer's needs

The information gathered reflected the hospital's philosophy of care based on the individual needs of patients. This was reinforced by a self-assessment form sent out to carers to enable them to state the patient's normal life-style and any problems they experienced in caring. A series of assumptions were made based on the analysis of previous care and research reports from the nursing and social literature that indicated the needs of carers. The assumptions are reflected through the range of outcome criteria discussed later in this chapter.

The assessment form was constructed from the six fundamental questions that constitute a preliminary assessment in Betty Neuman's model of nursing (Pearson and Vaughan, 1986) and from Freeman and Heinrich's Family Coping Index 1981 (cited by Turton and Orr, 1985). As with many other models of nursing, Betty Neuman bases assumptions about nursing on a wide range of knowledge drawn from physiology, sociology and psychology. An assumption can be described as knowledge that has not been established or tested, and a criticism which has been made of nursing models is that their theoretical assumptions have remained, in most cases, untested in practice. However, the Family Coping Index was empirically constructed following analysis of case study material. A draft assessment was tested to 'get it right' and to establish validity, that is to ensure that 'it does the job it was designed to do.' The use and analysis of this self-assessment tool is an example of a practice situation which can lead to the development of a theoretical framework (including an analysis of existing theoretical frameworks), which is subsequently returned to practice, tested, and shown to be valid using a retrospective case study approach.

1.8 Nursing knowledge of carer's needs (resource file)

The relevant knowledge concerning patients' and carers' needs was kept in a resource file, enabling easy access for the nurses as it was needed.

1.9 Patient always assigned to the same primary nurse

This criterion is based on the assumption that continuity of care, a key element in the theory of primary nursing (Manthey, 1980) is desirable. Whether patients prefer care based on this assumption is problematic and remains untested, the literature evaluating primary nursing being equivocal. However, my 'gut feeling' is that carers prefer this approach and gut feelings need to be recognized as significant sources of knowledge. They are not conjured up from nowhere, but reflect an accumulation of experience and insight. Benner (1984) draws an analogy of gut feelings with *gestalt*, the idea of seeing the situation as a whole with the parts becoming evident only later. In this respect many practice situations are gestalts which can be analysed later so that criteria which represent the parts can be identified.

Process criteria

The process criteria are written in terms of action. They are about doing things to achieve defined goals. These criteria generally reflect the structural knowledge previously discussed. This raises a distinction between structural knowledge, which enables people to make good decisions about situations, and what is generally referred to in nursing as practical skills, or the ability to do something in a skilful manner. In many instances nurses are unable to articulate their reasons for doing something or choosing an action, although they are skilled in the actual task. Similarly, nurses may have a good theoretical understanding of a situation but have difficulty with using this knowledge in practice. It seems that the traditional apprenticeship system of nurse training has not helped nurses to link these aspects of knowledge. Miller (1985) has described the difficulties that practical nurses face with getting access to knowledge about their practice, emphasizing the gap between theory and practice in nursing. Gould (1986) gives the particular example of pressure sore treatment and prevention and illustrates some reasons why nurses have difficulty with utilizing research that has been undertaken in this area of care. Argyris and Schon (1974) describe the difference between theories-of-action and theories-in-use. Theories-of-action is what somebody says they would do in a given situation, whereas theories-in-use are what they actually do. They claim the effective practitioner is the person whose theory-of-action matches theory-in-use, which reflects an appropriate level of knowledge.

Commentary

Criterion 2.3 suggests that the nurse should visit the patient and carer at home prior to first admission. Carers often used this time to inform the patient that respite care has been arranged. Where patients had expressed reluctance to accept respite care prior to the visit, it was often the time when they became sufficiently reassured to give their consent. It was also found that this visit enabled a 'breakdown of pretences' between the patient and carer, particularly where the relationship was marital. It helped to reassure the patient about the admission, and the carer about a perceived failure of duty. This value of home visits, although considered probable, was checked out through retrospective analysis. Visiting a carer and patient in their home when there is likelihood of a tense environment emphasizes the interpersonal aspects of skilled performance that may be needed by the nurse.

Criterion 2.5 states that the nurse uses the assessment form as the basis for discussion of care. It was assumed that this process would help to involve the carer in the hospital care process, thus recognizing his or her role as principal carer and providing reassurance that the patient's individual needs had at least been recognized, and hopefully would be met. This should help to develop trust between carer and nurse, leaving the carer with a sense of being in control and feeling confident about the patient's stay in hospital. These outcomes are recognized in the outcome criteria, demonstrating the relationship between different types of criteria. Trust has been shown to be a major factor in patients' and relatives' satisfaction with care (Thorne and Robinson, 1988). This was a significant source of knowledge in relation to outcome criterion 3.6: that is, that the carer would indicate satisfaction with care.

Outcome criteria

These criteria collectively reflect the practice situation and cover two fundamental elements:

- The organization of respite care
- The quality of respite care.

Criterion 3.1 reflects the organizational element and is easily ascertained. Over a period of time it would be possible to calculate what percentage of known people who would benefit from respite care received it on demand. Such knowledge can contribute to demonstrating the effectiveness of the organization.

The remaining criteria reflect the quality of the care received. They are assumptions based on a 'cocktail' derived from the literature, some of which has a research base (although very limited); the philosophy of care for the hospital, which reflected both the role of the hospital in helping people to remain in the community and being responsive to the community's needs; and experience of working with respite patients and their carers.

With reference to outcome criterion 3.5, the assessment form is used as a basis for discussion of care and recognizes the carer's principal role, a role in jeopardy with the perceived 'giving up' of care and associated failure of duty. Dawson (1987) has indicated a synonymous relationship between the marital role and the caring role, which can lead to feelings of guilt associated with accepting respite care. Monitoring the outcome criteria through case studies supports this research.

The assumptions reflected within the outcome criteria are also monitored to determine their validity. This, however, assumes the validity of the monitoring tools designed for this purpose. This issue introduces another source of knowledge, necessary for nurses in giving care, that can be developed in the process of writing and monitoring standards of care. Once standards have been monitored and results analysed, some prediction becomes possible for these outcomes. Checking out the validity of assumptions is part of a feedback process which may eventually change assumptions and lead to decisions being made on empirical evidence which should increase the effectiveness of care. The relationship between these factors is shown diagrammatically in figure 10.2.

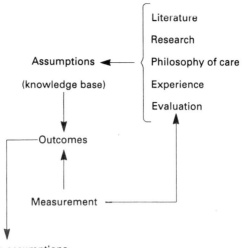

Figure 10.2   Making and checking assumptions

Within Clarke's definition of a nursing action, outcome criteria reflect what is beneficial for patients and their carers. The commentary on the structure, process and outcome criteria has identified the various sources of knowledge which contribute to this practice situation of providing an effective respite care service to the local community within the resources available. The standard demonstrates the interplay of sources of knowledge which it is imperative to consider in planning services within any local health setting.

The writing of standards is a particular way in which nurses can make use of existing knowledge in their everyday work. Knowledge is continuously changing in the light of new research and new ways of thinking and feeling about health issues. Hence the use of knowledge in practice has to be dynamic, an intrinsic quality of standards because of the necessity for constant review. Through the process of monitoring standards, nurses will constantly be checking out and validating their assumptions about practice, and adding to the stock of empirical knowledge to support nursing practice.

The commentary on the various criteria identifies many sources of knowledge. Most have been found by reading literature in which the basic disciplines of psychology and sociology have been applied to nursing, social care or health, rather than reading and applying the basic psychological and social concepts to the practice situation.

Some suggest that nursing is not, in itself, a basic discipline but a field of knowledge derived from other disciplines. However, nursing, as a practice discipline, draws on this knowledge in specific practice situations that are all intrinsically unique. The interplay of different sources of knowledge can never be the same, reflecting the uniqueness of each individual nurse, patient and carer, the relationship between them and the context of the local situation.

References

Argyris, C. and Schon, D.A. (1974) *Theory in Practice: Increasing Professional Effectiveness*, Jossey-Bass, San Francisco

Benner, P. (1984) *From Novice to Expert: Excellence and Power in Clinical Nursing*, Addison-Wesley, Menlo Park CA

Bergman, R. (1981) Accountability — definition and dimensions. *International Nursing Review*, **28(2)**, 53–58

Buckenham, J. and McGrath, G. (1983) *The Social Reality of Nursing*, Adis, Sydney

Clarke, M. (1986) Action and reflection: practice and theory in nursing. *Journal of Advanced Nursing*, **11**, 3–11

Dawson, J. (1987) Evaluation of a community-based night sitter service. In *Research in the Nursing Care of Elderly People* (ed. P. Fielding), Wiley, Chichester, 87–106

Department of Health and Social Security (1975) *Community Hospitals: Their Role and Development*, HSC (IS) 75, HMSO, London

Donabedian, A. (1968) Promoting quality through evaluating the process of patient care. *Medical Care*, **6(3)**, 181–201

Freeman, R.B. and Heinrich, J. (1981) *Community Health Nursing Practice*, 2nd edn, W.B. Saunders, London

Friedson, E. (1970) *Professional Dominance*, Atherton, Chicago

Gould, D. (1986) Pressure sore prevention and treatment: an example of nurses' failure to implement research findings. *Journal of Advanced Nursing*, **11**, 389–394

Jourard, S. (1971) *The Transparent Self*, Van Nostrand, Norwalk, New Jersey

Kitson, A. (1986) Indicators of quality of nursing care — an alternative approach. *Journal of Advanced Nursing*, **11**, 133–144

Lane-Franklyn, B.L. (1974) *Patient Anxiety on Admission to Hospital*, Royal College of Nursing, London

MacGuire, J. and Newberry, S. (1984) A measure of need. *Senior Nurse*, **1**, 17

Manthey, M. (1980) *The Practice of Primary Nursing*, Blackwell, Boston MA

Menzies, I.E.P. (1960) A case study in the functioning of social systems as a defence against anxiety. *Human Relations*, **13**, 95–120

Miller, A. (1985) The relationship between nursing theory and nursing practice. *Journal of Advanced Nursing*, **10**, 417–424

Pearson, A. and Vaughan, B. (1986) *Nursing Models for Practice*, Heinemann, London

Stein, L. (1978) The doctor–nurse game. In *Readings in Sociology of Nursing* (eds R. Dingwall and J. McIntosh), Churchill Livingstone, Edinburgh

Stockwell, F. (1972) *The Unpopular Patient*, Royal College of Nursing, London

Tucker, H. (1987) *The Role and Function of Community Hospitals*, project paper 70, Kings Fund, London

Turton, P. and Orr, J. (1985) *Learning to Care in the Community*, Hodder and Stoughton, London

Webster, D. (1985) Medical students' views of the nurse. *Nursing Research*, **34(5)**, 313–317

Chapter 11

Learning nursing knowledge

Philip Burnard

In this chapter some of the implications for nurse education of the teaching and learning of nursing knowledge are considered. It is useful to think of the process of learning about nursing in four stages. These are:

- The aims of nurse education
- The content of nurse education
- The methods of teaching and learning
- The assessment and evaluation of nurse education.

The chapter closes with an illustration of how the concepts under discussion can be applied in practice.

The aims of nurse education

What are the aims of nurse education? To train the nursing student to become an effective practitioner? To encourage the personal growth of the nurse? To provide a knowledge and skills base for the new entrant to the profession? Many more could probably be listed. Whilst it is essential that certain basic skills are learned by all nurses, it quickly becomes apparent that nurses work in very different situations, with very many different client groups. It is also apparent from the nursing literature that nursing knowledge is in a constant state of change. Two things follow from these factors:

- One type of training and educational process will not suit all groups of nursing students,
- Learning in nursing must be *lifelong*. We cannot hope to learn all we need in one course, nor even in a series of

courses. Nursing knowledge (like all types of knowledge) is developing and changing so rapidly that we must all be committed to learning throughout our careers.

Nursing education is thus a process of continually questioning and appraising what we know. Having said that, it is clear, too, that all nurses need to follow some formal programmes. It is therefore important to have basic diploma courses, followed by undergraduate and graduate programmes.

It is not sufficient, then, only to be committed to lifelong education. We must also be committed to the organization and management of structured courses. What must *not* happen, however, is that courses of this nature are allowed to ossify. We have probably all come across programmes which are running the same way now as they were five years ago. If it is true that nursing knowledge is constantly changing, then training and education must also change to reflect that progress. As we shall see, this has implications for both the content of formal educational programmes and for the methods of teaching and learning.

How then shall aims of courses be established? Traditionally, nurse educators were responsible for writing and publishing a series of aims and objectives for a given programme. These were usually known well in advance of students arriving for the course, and often known some *years* before the course started. Again, given the march of progress, such a situation seems far from ideal. So this begs the question: 'How else could things be done?'

Firstly, *some* aims are essential. To set up a course at all is to have certain motives in mind and to have some idea of what the 'product' may be. Just as students do not come to courses as 'blank slates', nor do nurse educators plan courses with no end-point in mind. In recent years, there has been much discussion about student-centred learning (Rogers, 1983; Burnard and Chapman, 1990). Sometimes, this notion of student-centredness has led to the idea that *no* course planning should take place and that students should be left to decide what it is they want to learn. In nursing, and particularly in preregistration courses, such a situation is inadequate. Nurses who are required to register as competent in a certain set of skills must learn those skills. We cannot assume that all nurses will 'naturally' choose to learn them and there are times when the leaders of courses are much more clear about the learning goals than the students.

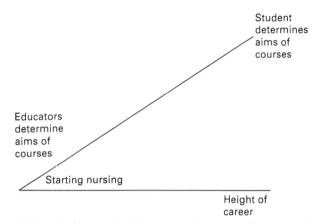

Figure 11.1   Relationship between educational aims and who determines them

In postgraduate studies, however, the situation is different. Here, the nurse has already gained certain required attributes and learned the necessary skills and basic knowledge. The postgraduate can then choose the field of knowledge or skills that he or she wants to pursue in greater depth. Arguably, such students *should* negotiate their own programmes. In a sense, only they know what they need to know next.

It is possible to note a changing set of relationships between educators and students. In the early part of the process of becoming a nurse, courses are highly structured and the aims clearly spelt out. As the process continues, the student comes more and more to determine his or her own learning needs and wants. Figure 11.1 illustrates this changing relationship.

The content of nurse education

What is there to learn about nursing? The question is one that raises epistemological issues. Epistemology is the philosophy of knowledge. It is concerned with how we *know* things. Earlier in this book, Carper's (1978) patterns of knowledge in nursing were discussed. This chapter offers a threefold typology of knowledge that can also be applied to nursing. Three types of knowledge that go towards the make up of an individual may be described as propositional knowledge, practical knowledge and experiential knowledge (Heron, 1981).

Propositional knowledge

Propositional knowledge is that which may be contained in theories or models. It may be described as 'textbook' knowledge and is synonymous with Ryle's (1949) concept of 'knowing that', which is a concept further developed in an educational context by Pring (1976). A person may build up a considerable bank of facts, theories or ideas about a subject, person or thing, without necessarily having any direct experience of that subject, person or thing. A person, may, for example, develop a considerable propositional knowledge about, say, midwifery, without ever necessarily having been anywhere near a woman who is having a baby! Presumably it would be more useful to combine that knowledge with some practical experience, but this does not necessarily have to be the case. This, then, is the domain of propositional knowledge. Obviously it is possible to have propositional knowledge about a great number of subject areas, ranging from science to literature or from counselling to physiology. Any information contained in books must necessarily be of the propositional sort.

Nurses have developed a wide range of propositional knowledge about nursing theories and models. What is essential to the development of such propositional knowledge is critical thinking and research. We need to be able to reflect on knowledge and remain open to its revision. To lose the ability to think critically is to stagnate. At best, it is to accept that what other people say is 'correct' in some way. The critical approach is as vital in nursing as it is in any other discipline. Until recently, nurses have not been encouraged to take a critical approach to dealing with knowledge. Research is also vital here. It is the means of testing out some theories and models with the 'real world'. It is one thing to have a model of how things work or how people are. It is quite another to test out the validity of that model with real life. If we do not constantly check theorizing with the way the world *actually* is, we always run the risk of confusing the model with the world itself. We come to believe that our model not only represents real life but *is* real life (Claxton, 1984).

Practical knowledge

Practical knowledge is knowledge developed through the acquisition of skills. Thus, changing a dressing or driving a motor cycle demonstrates practical knowledge, though,

equally, so does the use of counselling skills which involve the use of specific verbal and non-verbal behaviours and intentional use of counselling interventions as described above. Pract-
ical knowledge is synonymous with Ryle's (1949) concept of 'knowing how', which was developed in an educational context by Pring (1976). Usually more than mere 'knack', practical knowledge is the substance of a smooth performance of a practical or interpersonal skill. A considerable amount of a nurses's time is taken up with the demonstration of practical knowledge – often, but not always, of the interpersonal sort.

Like propositional knowledge, our practical knowledge needs constant updating. The need for certain skills passes. New skills are developed. The person who is committed to lifelong education appreciates that skills are not a 'once and for all' thing but a perpetual process of developing, refining and changing.

Most educational programmes in schools and colleges have concerned themselves primarily with both propositional and practical knowledge, but particularly the former. Thus the 'propositional knowledge' aspect of a person is the aspect that is often held in highest regard. Practical knowledge, although respected, is usually seen as slightly less important than the propositional sort. In nursing, an interesting split has occurred. Whilst those who work in the clinical setting tend to prize practical knowledge above any other, those in educational settings seem more concerned with propositional knowledge. The knack is to try to develop both in tandem.

The proficient nurse is one who is both clinically skilled and academically able. He or she is interested in both practical work and in explanations of how or why such practical work is therapeutic. The two should be inextricably linked.

Experiential knowledge

Experiential knowledge is knowledge gained through direct encounter with a subject, person or thing. It is the subjective and affective nature of that encounter that contributes to this sort of knowledge. Experiential knowledge is knowledge through relationship. Such knowledge is synonymous with Roger's (1983) description of experiential learning and with Polanyi's concept of 'personal' knowledge and 'tacit' knowledge (Polanyi, 1958). On reflection it may appear that most of the things that are really important to us belong in this

domain. If personal relationships with other people are considered, it may be discovered that what we like or love about
them cannot be reduced to a series of propositional statements,
and yet the feelings we have for them are vital and part of
what is most important in our lives. Most encounters with
others contain the possible seeds of experiential knowledge. It
is only when we are so detached from other people that we
treat them as objects that no experiential learning can occur
(except learning how to treat people as objects!). An important
aim in nursing relationships must be to continue to learn more
about people as changing, vulnerable and individual human
beings.

That does not mean that all experiential knowledge is tied
exclusively to relationships with other people. For example, I
had propositional knowledge about the United States before
I went there. When I went there, all that propositional
knowledge was changed considerably. What I had known was
changed by my direct experience of the country. I had
developed *experiential* knowledge of the place. Experiential
knowledge is not of the same type or order as propositional or
practical knowledge. It is, nevertheless, critical, in that it
affects everything else we think about or do.

Experiential knowledge is necessarily personal and idiosyncratic. Indeed, as Rogers (1983) points out, it may be difficult
to convey to another person in words. Words tend to be loaded
with personal (often experiential) meanings, and thus to
understand each other we need to understand the nature of
the way in which the people with whom we converse use
words. It is arguable, however, that such experiential knowledge is sometimes conveyed to others through gesture, eye
contact, tone of voice, inflection and all the other non-verbal
and paralinguistic aspects of communication (Arnold and
Boggs, 1989). Indeed, it may be experiential knowledge that is
passed on when two people (for example a nurse and patient)
become very involved with each other in a conversation, a
learning encounter or counselling.

The methods of teaching and learning

If there are different types of knowledge, it follows that there
will also be different ways of gaining that knowledge. We
cannot learn experiential knowledge from a lecture any more
than we can gain an understanding of a nursing model from

skills training. Different types of knowledge call for different kinds of learning method. The accent here is on *learning*. Most educational programmes up until recent times have been concerned with *teaching*. If we change the accent, we change the emphasis away from formal, classroom teaching sessions and return the responsibility for learning to the learner. As we noted in the first part of this chapter, learning is a lifelong process. We cannot afford to stay dependent on teachers and lecturers for our learning needs. Each one of us needs to become an independent learner. Again, if we consider Figure 11.1, we will note that it is possible to move from dependence on teaching staff for organizing and structuring our learning towards independent learning activities in which we determine and fulfil our own learning needs.

What learning methods are at our disposal? It may be useful to consider the three types of knowledge, propositional, practical and experiential, in order to answer that question. It was noted earlier that propositional knowledge is concerned with theories and models. Thus the learning methods that are identifiable here are lectures, reading and the more formal approaches to learning. Practical knowledge, on the other hand, is concerned with skills, both psychomotor and interpersonal. This sort of knowledge can be learned through skills training, through observing role models and through trying out new behaviours. A useful combination of methods is first to attend formal skills training and then to try out the new skills in real life situations. It is then possible to monitor and adapt the skills learned in the training setting. Such a process involves the learner in reflecting on his or her performance in the real setting and perhaps inviting colleagues and friends to offer feedback.

Interpersonal skills can often be learned through experiential learning methods (Heron, 1982; Burnard, 1989a, 1990). These can be most easily described as methods that involve 'learning by doing'. We cannot, for example, learn how to counsel another person through being lectured on the topic. We can learn to counsel through practising counselling skills with another person.

The experiential knowledge domain opens up greater challenges. How do we 'learn' experiential knowledge? To learn experientially is to learn more about ourselves: our skills, values, beliefs, attitudes and so on. The key to learning in the experiential domain is *reflection*. We noted above that reflection was an important part of learning interpersonal skills. It is *vital* in the field of experiential knowledge. In order to learn more about ourselves we need first to learn to reflect on what we do. This means that we must be able to consciously *notice* what we think and feel as we think and feel. There are various learning tools which can help here. First, the use of a reflective diary. Such a diary remains private to the individual but is one in which the nurse can note down his or her thoughts, feelings and changing attitudes. The diary can aid reflection on the process of change, both as it occurs and after it has occurred. It enables nurses to look back and review their progress in the experiential domain. Also, because they are required to write in it regularly, it encourages the development of the reflective approach as a way of life.

A second approach to exploring experiential knowledge is via a small group that meets for such a purpose. The experiential group is one that gets together with the aim of reflecting on practice and sharing viewpoints. All that is required here is that each member is prepared to listen to the others, share his or her experiences and thoughts and remain open-minded. Such groups can meet in educational or clinical settings and can be led by anyone who is prepared to remain appreciative of the fact that there is no 'right' answer to anything and who is mature enough to respect views different from his or her own.

The assessment and evaluation of nurse education

These are two separate issues which are often confused with each other. As a general rule, *people* are assessed for their knowledge or skill level. *Courses* are evaluated. How, then, do we assess our levels of skill and knowledge in nursing? Sometimes, the question is answered for us. Most formal training and educational courses have examination and assessment procedures built in. Such procedures are usually not negotiable. You either pass the examinations or you fail the course. Increasingly, though, course developers are including aspects of *self-assessment* in nursing courses. What does such self-assessment involve?

First, it requires that all participants are clear about personal aims and goals. We cannot assess how far we have come unless we know what we are aiming for. In self-assessment, then, it is useful to have some personal goals identified at the beginning of a course or workshop. Many nurse educators are moving towards the notion of the learning contract (Knowles,

1975). With the learning contract, personal objectives or goals are determined by the individual at the beginning of a course and serve as guideposts throughout that course. At the end of the learning encounter they can serve two purposes. First, they can help the individual to identify what he or she has learned. Second, they can help determine the *next* stage in the learning process. Here, again, we see the need for lifelong education. Of course no formal course can take us to the target of learning. We always need to be looking ahead to the next course or the next set of learning goals.

Course evaluation leads to another set of issues. How are courses evaluated and what is done once such evaluation has taken place? The most formal forms of course evaluation involve prepared questionnaires which course leaders hand out to participants at the end of a course or workshop. The advantages of such an approach are clear. Questionnaires are easy to administer and check. Their drawback is that they tend to lack personal involvement and can be seen as a chore by those filling them in. Also, the whole process can degenerate into a paper exercise: the questionnaires are filled in, the results duly recorded and nothing else happens.

An alternative approach is that which involves reflection and discussion. At the end of a course, participants are invited to divide into pairs or small groups and to reflect on the course. They then identify the parts of the course that they *did* and *did not* find useful. This is followed by a plenary session in which all participants feed back their likes and dislikes. After this feedback session, participants are invited to make suggestions as to how the next course could be modified. All of the comments and suggestions are noted by the course leader who can then incorporate them into the planning stage of the next course. This method has the advantages of spontaneity and personal involvement, although it may lack the more formal rigour of the questionnaire approach.

Personal change and development

So far this chapter has explored some of the issues in developing nursing knowledge. It has considered the question of the aims of nurse education and of who sets those aims. It has considered different types of nursing knowledge. There has also been a discussion of various approaches to learning, assessing and evaluating. The accent, throughout, has been on learning in nursing being a lifelong process. However, there is often a large gap between thinking and doing. If we are really committed to change and to continuing our own educational processes, action must occur. We must go further than just identifying our needs and wants. We must lay out a practical plan of development. Friere (1972) has called this process 'praxis'. The process of reflection and action can be a useful one, both for ourselves and for the colleagues with whom we work. The stages of the process are easily identified:

- *Stage 1*: reflection on the current state of knowledge and skills
- *Stage 2*: the drawing up of an action plan
- *Stage 3*: the putting of the plan into action
- *Stage 4*: reflection on the outcome.

This set of stages can develop into a cycle of events. As we work through the stages we constantly check our knowledge and skills base against two things: our own needs and wants and the needs and wants determined by the job that we do. If these two domains of working, the personal and the professional, could be kept together it could ensure that nurse education is constantly updated and enhanced. Thus nursing knowledge may be added to through discussion, research and publication.

The experiential curriculum: teaching counselling in the nursing curriculum – a case in point

It is important to consider how the concepts in this chapter 'work' in practice and an example may help here. Under discussion is the teaching and learning of counselling skills in a nursing education programme. Figure 11.2 illustrates an experiential curriculum model. The four stages of the model are: (1) a theory input; (2) practice of skills; (3) application of the skills learned; and (4) evaluation of learning and identification of new goals. Underpinning and supporting all of these stages is the notion of reflection, and this reflection is the core feature of the learning process. We have two choices in life: we can either let things happen to us and not notice them or we can reflect on what happens and learn from the process. Thus, reflection is important during the theory input, the practice aspect, the application of skills and during the evaluation period.

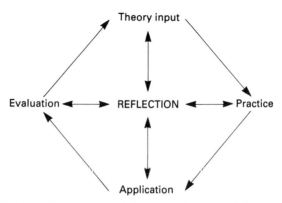

Figure 11.2   An experiential curriculum model

How does the experiential curriculum link with the types of knowledge discussed in this chapter? First, in the theory input (stage 1), students are offered propositional knowledge in the form of theories of counselling, 'maps' of the counselling relationship and a rationale for the use of counselling in nursing (Nelson-Jones, 1981; Tschudin, 1986; Burnard, 1989b). Second, in the practice stage (stage 2), students practise a range of counselling skills and thus develop practical knowledge. The experiential learning methods discussed above are useful here.

Next (stage 3), they apply those two types of knowledge in the clinical setting, either in the hospital or community. Through this 'real life' experience, those students gain experiential knowledge. They extend their range of counselling skills and also learn more about themselves and other people in the process. In the evaluation stage (stage 4), those three types of knowledge are compared and contrasted and new learning objectives are drawn up. During this stage, the students determine whether or not they need more propositional, practical or experiential knowledge (or, perhaps, a combination of all three). In this stage they work through the process described, above, in the discussion on 'reflection and action'.

Figure 11.3 illustrates the complete curriculum model and its relationship with the three forms of knowledge. At times in such a curriculum there will be an overlap of the different sorts of knowledge. An understanding of the three types can, however, enable both students and educational staff to analyse new learning needs and identify educational opportunities.

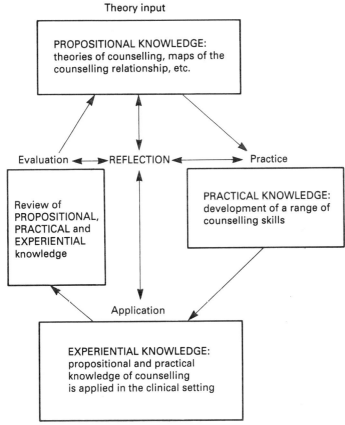

Figure 11.3   The experiential curriculum in practice

The types may also ensure that there is a balance in the curriculum between theoretical knowledge on the one hand and practical and experiential knowledge on the other.

The emphasis on counselling in this illustration is merely by way of example. The model described here can be used to teach a wide range of practical nursing and interpersonal skills and can be adapted for use either in the college or the clinical setting. It has been used by the author to teach a range of interpersonal skills to nurses at diploma, undergraduate and graduate level and in continuing nurse education. There is no reason to suppose that all of the theory input must take place in the college of nursing; it could just as easily be imparted by clinical practitioners.

This chapter has offered another epistemological approach to nursing knowledge and demonstrated how that approach can be used in practice, via an experiential curriculum model. Such a model honours not only the propositional knowledge of textbooks but also the practical and experiential knowledge developed out of the practice of nursing.

References

Arnold, E. and Boggs, K. (1989) *Interpersonal Relationships: Professional Communication Skills for Nurses*, W.B. Saunders, Philadelphia

Burnard, P. (1989a) *Teaching Interpersonal Skills: A Handbook of Experiential Learning for Health Professionals*, Chapman and Hall, London

Burnard, P. (1989b) *Counselling Skills for Health Professionals*, Chapman and Hall, London

Burnard, P. (1990) *Learning Human Skills*, 2nd edn, Butterworth-Heinemann, Oxford

Burnard, P. and Chapman, C. (1990) *Nurse Education: The Way Forward*, Scutari, London

Carper, B.A. (1978) Fundamental patterns of knowing in nursing. *Advances in Nursing Science*, **1 (1)**, 13–23

Claxton, G. (1984) *Live and Learn*, Harper and Row, London

Friere, P. (1972) *Pedagogy of the Oppressed*, Penguin, London

Heron, J. (1981) Philosophical basis for a new paradigm. In P. Reason and J. Rowan *Human Inquiry: A Sourcebook of New Paradigm Research* (eds P. Reason and J. Rowan), Wiley, Chichester, pp. 19–35

Heron, J. (1982) *Experiential Training Techniques*, 2nd edn, Human Potential Research Project, University of Surrey, Guildford

Knowles, M. (1975) *Self-Directed Learning*, Cambridge Books, New York

Nelson-Jones, R. (1981) *The Theory and Practice of Counselling Psychology*, Holt, Rinehart and Winston, New York

Polanyi, M. (1958) *Personal Knowledge*, University Press, Chicago

Pring, R. (1976) *Knowledge and Schooling*, Basic Books, London

Rogers, C.R. (1983) *Freedom to Learn for the Eighties*, Merrill, Columbus OH

Ryle, G. (1949) *The Concept of Mind*, Peregrine, London

Tschudin, V. (1986) *Counselling Skills for Nurses*, Baillière Tindall, London

Part Four

Future Issues

In this final section of the book we have brought together three different, and each in their own way, radical commentaries to complement earlier readings and stimulate further debate. The chapters are idiosyncratic in nature, expressing the very personal views of the authors. Hence, each one has been written in the first person rather than the more traditional style of using third person which has been adhered to earlier in the text.

Chapters 12 and 13 cover areas which impinge on nursing although they are not directly concerned with 'knowing' nursing itself. However, it has to be remembered that the context in which nursing takes place will inevitably influence the way in which nursing is practised. That we work in an era where the use of technology is dominant and will impinge on our everyday working lives cannot be denied. What becomes critical then is that the use of technology becomes our slave rather than our master. In Chapter 12, Hugh Robinson offers words of caution and highlights the danger of becoming bemused by the cumulated data which modern systems can help us to store. While the values of these systems cannot be denied, the danger of failing to differentiate between information and knowledge could lead nurses into stormy seas. Learning to master the systems and take advantage of what they can offer is crucial in this day and age, but expertise is also needed to use the information wisely, never denying the context in which it was gathered.

Many nurses have suggested that politics are not for them; that nurses, in their caring roles, need not concern themselves with either local or national political matters. However, in Chapter 13 Kate Robinson argues that life is not that simple and that the influence of external forces on everyday practice is there for all to see. It can be suggested that it is only the naïve who consider that politics are not relevant to them; some of the influencing factors are explored in this chapter.

In Chapter 14, Alan Pearson offers a personal view of the emerging paradigms which are coming to light in the world of nursing. His views are clear and powerful in seeing the future role which nurses could play in the total health care service.

Perhaps they offer a challenge to each one of us to look at the ways in which we can contribute to the development of the discipline of nursing.

We hope you will find the views offered in this section of the book thought-provoking. Some of the ideas may seem unfamiliar on first reading and may need to be returned to at a later date. Indeed, this is a comment which applies to many parts of the book. However, the importance of taking count of a wide range of ideas, views and perspectives can undoubtedly enhance the understanding of nurses in their everyday practice, helping to open their eyes to the potential of nursing for the future.

Chapter 12

The mechanization of knowledge

Hugh Robinson

> For it was the Rabbi Löw who constructed the many-legended
> robot-figure of the Golem, which he could secretly endow with
> life by opening its mouth and inserting slips of paper on which
> magic formulae were inscribed.
>
> Patrick Leigh Fermor, *A Time of Gifts*

In this chapter, I want to examine some issues that arise with
the representation and processing of knowledge through technological systems, in particular that of computer technology.
These issues are important in any account of the epistemology
of nursing for two related reasons.

The first reason is straightforward and brutally empirical:
increasingly, nurses are faced with the practical problem of
responding to the use of computer technology in their everyday professional lives. How does a nurse respond to the glow of
a visual display unit (VDU) screen and the chatter of a printer
when these two pieces of hardware are mechanically driven by
some patient-care planning software (which, like all software,
appears to be mystifyingly intangible) and are producing
output that recommends a particular form of patient care for a
particular patient in his or her charge? The computer system
makes the recommendation and lays claim to the authority of
knowledge. Is this knowledge entirely equivalent to that of a
senior nurse giving the same recommendation? In what ways
might it differ? These are practical problems for *nurses* to solve
but, to aid that solution, it is helpful to understand the ways in
which computer technology constrains and transforms knowledge. This chapter is a contribution to that necessary understanding.

The second reason for considering the representation and processing of knowledge by computer technology is concerned with influencing the curriculum of nurse education. It is generally agreed that some attention is paid in the curriculum to computer technology, yet it is unclear as to exactly what that attention should be. One approach is that of teaching some appreciation of the mechanics of the technology. So, nurses grapple with the distinction between hardware and software, learn to tell their bits from their bytes, and know when they need a hard disk rather than a floppy one. This chapter considers such teaching as being inappropriate, in the sense that nurse education needs to consider *what* computer technology does, rather than *how* it does it. An alternative (and somewhat more appropriate) approach, which is sometimes taken, is that of considering the impact of computer technology under the broad heading of *the social implications of computer technology*, or some similar rubric. Such an approach assumes that the technology is neutral. That is to say, there is the belief that computer technology itself is neither a 'good' thing nor a 'bad' thing. Instead, an emphasis is laid on how the technology is used, in particular applications and circumstances, as being the thing that may be 'good' or 'bad'. However, this approach is still by no means adequate and this chapter challenges the presumption of technological neutrality and argues that computer technology brings with it a particular view of the world by virtue of its construction and representation of knowledge, irrespective of the particular applications and circumstances of its use. Specifically, current computer technology regards knowledge as being capable of being codified, measured and governed by rules. This, as much as anything else, is the very stuff of what computers do.

Technologies of information

The term *information* has not been used frequently in previous chapters. Here, however, I want to regard it simply as knowledge in a purposeful guise; information being any form of communication that provides understandable and useful knowledge for the person receiving it. What then of *information technology?* A useful working definition of information technology is that it is the processing, representation and transmission of information by means of technology. Information technology does not consist of a single technology: rather, it is a range of technologies utilized together in a way that varies with situation. For example, use of a cash card involves at least three different technologies. First, there is the electromechanical technology that physically manipulates the plastic card within the cash point machine and electronically reads the necessary details from the card. Second, there is the telecommunications technology that transmits the details of the request to the bank's computer system and, hopefully, the computer's authorization back to the cash point machine. Third, there is the computer technology that maintains the details of each customer's bank account and records the fact that a debit has been made in the appropriate account.

In this chapter, I shall not attempt to cover all the constituent technologies of information technology. Instead, I concentrate on the representation and processing of knowledge through computer technology – the technology of one of the dominant machines of the modern world. To illustrate the issues raised, I shall consider three paradigms for the use of computer technology. (I use paradigm here in its mundane sense and not in the specific sense developed by Kuhn, 1970.) The *first* paradigm is that of knowledge as data and is characterized by computer database systems, such as those used to support patient record systems. The *second* paradigm is that of knowledge as processing and is characterized by computer systems that carry out various calculations, such as statistical analysis systems. The *third*, and final paradigm, is that of knowledge as rules and is characterized by so-called 'expert systems'.

Data and knowledge

The first paradigm to be considered emphasizes the ability of computer technology to store and retrieve large quantities of data. I will argue that this paradigm constrains and transforms knowledge in a number of significant ways: it introduces a distinction between information (knowledge) and data, it regards knowledge as homogeneous and capable of being structured and codified, and it encourages the view that knowledge consists of facts about a reality which endures outside of any social context. To be sure, the paradigm also enables certain forms of knowledge to be made available in a way which hitherto has not been possible.

123	364	747
Mrs Joan Duncombe	Mr Mohamed Khan	Miss Jane Maier
F	M	F
14 Seamark St	74 Clarks Rd	2 Water Lane
Ledbury	Monmouth	Upper Slaughter
Herefordshire	Gwent	Gloucestershire
D	M	S
060956	140342	240579
4451	6675	4451

Figure 12.1   Three patient records

In making these arguments, it is convenient to use a specific example and to these ends a patient record system will be used. The system records details of the patients who are being treated in hospital, including the wards they are on, the nurses responsible for their nursing treatment, the doctors responsible for their medical treatment, the drugs they have been prescribed, and so on. Typically a (computer) record is held for each patient, as well as records for each ward, doctor, nurse and drug. The collection of all such records constitutes the **database** for the system (see Robinson, 1989, for further technical details). I shall concentrate on just the records that relate to patients. Here, in Figure 12.1, are three examples of a (much simplified) patient record, as they might be stored by the system.

Figure 12.1 immediately illustrates an important point about this first paradigm: the technology stores *data*; it does not store *information*. For example, whilst it may seem reasonable to assume that 'Mrs Joan Duncombe' is the name of a patient and that her address is '14 Seamark St, Ledbury, Herefordshire', it is not at all clear what '123', 'F', 'D', '060956', and '4451' mean in terms of the information about a patient. In order for these records to convey information, it is necessary to know the structure of a record and the intended meaning of the components in that structure. Figure 12.2 gives the structure of a patient record and its relation to the records for Mrs Duncombe and Mr Khan.

PATIENT NUMBER	123	364
NAME	Mrs Joan Duncombe	Mr Mohamed Khan
SEX	F	M
ADDRESS	14 Seamark St	74 Clarks Rd
	Ledbury	Monmouth
	Herefordshire	Gwent
MARITAL STATUS	D	M
DATE OF BIRTH	060956	140342
NURSE	4451	6675

Figure 12.2   The structure of a patient record

Thus, Mrs Duncombe has a PATIENT NUMBER of '123', a SEX of 'F', a MARITAL STATUS of 'D', a DATE OF BIRTH of '060956' and a NURSE of '4451'. Furthermore, the meaning of each component in the structure (PATIENT NUMBER, NAME, SEX, ADDRESS, MARITAL STATUS, DATE OF BIRTH and NURSE) needs to be known and agreed upon. For example, it needs to be known that the PATIENT NUMBER is a reference number that uniquely identifies each patient, since there will be instances of two or more patients having the same name (there may be several patients whose name is Mohamed Khan, for example). Similarly, it needs to be known that the NURSE component contains the staff number identifying the nurse responsible for the patient's nursing treatment. The meaning of the coded values in a field also need to be known, for example that a MARITAL STATUS of 'D' means divorced and 'M' means married. To be pedantic, it also needs to be known that a DATE OF BIRTH value of '060956' means 6th September 1956, as opposed to June 9th 1956, which is how nurse in the USA would interpret those six digits.

Given the structure and intended meaning of the components of a record, the data stored may be interpreted as recording certain facts about a patient: that the patient identified by 123 is Mrs Joan Duncombe, who is female and lives at 14 Seamark St, Ledbury, Herefordshire; she is divorced and was born on 6th September 1956; she is nursed by the nurse identified by 4451. The record for Mr Khan needs to be interpreted in a similar fashion, as does the record for Miss Maier. Indeed, *all* patient records need to be interpreted in this fashion: the structure and intended meaning of the components applies to any patient record. The technology of structured, formatted and codified records does not permit anything but minor variations between individual records and, as a consequence, regards knowledge as being necessarily homogeneous and capable of being codified.

To take the issue of homogeneity first: the facts that constitute knowledge of a patient have the same form for each patient. That is to say, all patients have names, are of determinant sex and of fixed abode, have clear marital status and known date of birth, and have their nursing care allocated to a known nurse. The absence of any one of these facts for a particular patient is, of course, allowed. For example, a patient's exact date of birth may not be known, since, say, the patient's ethnic background is one where no great significance is placed on remembering such details. However, the absence of a fact for a patient, such as a date of birth, is typically and simply recorded by the technology as 'missing information', thus reinforcing the standard of homogeneity. (Indeed, the technology itself finds such missing information aberrant and problematic; see Date, 1990, pp.384–388, for example.)

Similar problems are raised where there is a need to record *additional* information about an individual patient: it cannot easily be fitted into the standard record structure that must hold for all patients (see Kent, 1979, for an account of the technical issues associated with homogeneity). Typically, additional information may be recorded in an extra record component as some form of comment. As such, it is accorded a status subsidiary to the standard information recorded for a patient: that is to say, it is knowledge of a lower value than the standard 'knowledge'.

The codification of knowledge stems from the technology's need to select and retrieve records on the basis of discrete and testable values rather than on textual descriptions. The most obvious cases in the example of a patient record are of sex and marital status. The use of two codes, M and F, to denote sex may seem unproblematic since people (and patients) are of one sex or the other. Issues raised by sex change patients may seem pathological and bizarre, rather than being knowledge that cannot be recorded in a homogeneous and codified fashion. However, the case of marital status is more illuminating. Suppose the codes for marital status are 'D' (for divorced), 'M' (for married), 'S' (for single) and 'P' (for separated). Such a categorization and codification of marital status forces knowledge about a patient's marital status to be regarded as falling within these four categories. Knowledge such as the fact that Mrs Duncombe is divorced but has formed a stable, permanent and caring relationship with another partner cannot be recorded except, as before, in an extra component in the computer record given the name and status appropriate to 'comments'. Even this may not be possible and the facts about her marital status may take the form of written notes or verbal information communicated from nurse to nurse. Either way, Mrs Duncombe's marital status is recorded as being that of divorced and being on a par with all other patients who also have the marital status of divorced. This is not a problem that can be solved by extending the categorization and codification to cover marital status in a more discriminating fashion. Extending the coding system to cover all the subtle variations in the richness of personal relationships proves to be an unworkable task (see Robinson, 1986, pp.21–24, for a critique of categorization in the context of health visiting).

My final substantive point about this first paradigm concerns the way in which computer technology encourages a view that knowledge is knowledge of an objective reality. The technology records knowledge about patients in a way that views all patients as being essentially similar in their factual (that is, epistemological) structure and with many features of their everyday lives being amenable to categorization. As such, the mechanization of knowledge has introduced an abstraction away from a concern for individuals and their mundane differences. The 'facts' recorded about all patients are 'facts' placed outside their individual social contexts. They become facts about an enduring and objective reality. Typically, this can be seen in the way that the abstraction (the patient record system) is perceived as a neutral and objective statement of what is the case. For example, Mrs Duncombe is divorced not so much because of a major upheaval in her life or because of some legal process: she is divorced because she has a MARITAL STATUS of 'D'.

The general points that I have made above, via the example of a patient record system, should not be seen as a form of Luddite epistemology. (The Luddites were an early nineteenth century group of workers who responded to the introduction of labour saving machines in the textile industry by smashing the machines, on the grounds that they threatened their livelihood.) Without doubt, the use of computer technology in patient record systems confers significant advantages in terms of the efficiency and quality of the care that may be delivered. However, these advantages also bring with them, for better or worse, a transformation of knowledge in the manner I have outlined above. Mathiassen and Andersen (1983, p.255) describe the introduction of a computer system as effecting just such a transformation: 'the system invites a special concept of nursing and disease: from being based upon the speech acts of description and interpretation, it shifted towards classification and determination of species.'

This first paradigm emphasizes knowledge as being knowledge of what is the case: a knowledge of facts which the computer technology adroitly stores and retrieves. In a sense, no new knowledge is generated: the facts that are retrieved are facts which have been stored previously. In the next paradigm, that of knowledge as processing, the emphasis shifts to one where the technology transforms existing facts into new facts.

Processing and knowledge

A patient record system, such as that referred to in the previous section, will record information about patients, as I have outlined. It will also record information about wards, the beds they contain, and the period for which a patient occupies a particular bed. Given this information it is possible to calculate, by means of a simple computer program, the bed occupancy rate for a ward for a period of time. Thus, a particular ward might have a bed occupancy rate of 80% for January, meaning that the ward's beds were occupied 80% of the time during that month.

In a sense, again, no new knowledge is being produced: the computer program carries out processing which has merely added up each day's occupancy for each bed, over a month, and expressed the result as a percentage. The information (the knowledge) was always there, recorded on the database: it has been simply processed or summarized as a statistic. For example, if a ward has 20 beds and all these beds were available for use in a 30-day monthly accounting period, then a bed occupancy rate of 100% would be achieved if each of these beds were occupied by a patient on each day; that is, $20 \times 30 = 600$ bed days. However, suppose that the patient record system shows that the bed occupancy was, in fact, 500 bed days. This is known by examining the information held about each bed for each day in the 30-day accounting period. The bed occupancy rate is then $500 \div 600 \times 100 = 83.3333333\%$. This hardly seems to constitute the transformation of existing facts (600 available bed days, 500 actual bed days) into new facts (83.3333333%).

However, in an important sense, new knowledge has been produced and the (simple) processing of information constitutes a paradigm for the mechanization of knowledge. The very objective neutrality of the processing carried out on the input, the individual occupancy for each bed, confers an objective neutrality to the output that transcends its derived and calculated nature. The bed occupancy rate ceases to be a convenient and notional summary: it is reified into an objective and factual property of a ward (this is heightened by the spurious accuracy of seven decimal places conferred by the computation of an approximate real number.) This objective and factual nature stems also from its origins: the very standard and homogeneous facts of the previous section. Hence, a twofold process has taken place: facts about a (supposedly) enduring and objective reality have been processed to produce (new) objective and neutral facts.

Wards with differing bed occupancy rates are seen as wards that have different properties. A ward with a bed occupancy rate of 95% is different from a ward with a bed occupancy rate of 75% and, inevitably, this quantitative difference is viewed as a qualitative difference: a ward with a rate of 95% is 'better', in some sense, than a ward with a rate of 75%. A typical presumption would be that 'better' here means something akin to 'managed more effectively' or 'providing better value for money'.

Yet, of course, this supposed qualitative difference may be more apparent than real when the individual contexts of wards are taken into account. The 'better' ward (the 95% ward) may be 'hot bedding' patients or the 'less good' ward (the 75% ward) may, responsibly and professionally, be using some beds for planned respite care. Yet these contexts and circumstances now stand divorced from the objective and neutral measurement of knowledge: they are accorded a status subsidiary to the 'hard' measurement of knowledge enshrined in the bed occupancy rate. At best, these contexts and circumstances are seen as 'explanations' for objective states of affairs – why the rate is not as high as it should be – rather than the very stuff of nursing care and management.

As before, I would emphasize that I am not seeking to deny the benefits to be gained from this paradigm of knowledge as processing. The nature of these benefits, and the necessity for achieving them, have been vigorously pursued by NHS management (see Windsor, 1986, for example). Rather, I would seek merely to stress that such benefits also bring with them, for better or worse, a transformation of knowledge.

Rules and knowledge

I now turn to my final paradigm, that of knowledge as rules. In particular, I wish to examine the manifestation of computer technology known as the *expert system*. Simplistically, expert systems seek to enshrine, in computer software, the relevant (cognitive) behaviour of a human expert in some given problem area where the application of expertise is seen as appropriate. For example, the expert system MYCIN (Shortliffe, 1976) diagnoses bacterial infections in hospital patients, whereas the PLANT/cd system (Boulanger, 1983) predicts black cutworm damage to corn. Expert systems have yet to become as commonplace in nursing as the previous examples which I have used, but there is evidence that this process is changing (for example, see Jones, 1988; Massie, 1988; von Grey, 1990). So, by way of illustration, a patient assessment expert system would claim to mimic the patient assessment expertise of a nursing expert.

The claim of such expert systems to display expertise stems from the recording, in software, of knowledge in two ways. Firstly, there is the simple recording of *facts*. To take an example from the MYCIN domain of bacterial infection diagnosis, we might have the following three facts:

```
The stain of Sample 7 is grampos
The morphology of Sample 7 is coccus
The growth conformation of Sample 7 is chains
```

Or, to take a deliberately simple nursing example, we might have
the following two facts:

```
The patient in bed 7 is unconscious
The patient in bed 7 has no detectable pulse
```

Secondly, there is the recording of *rules*, such as, in the case of MYCIN:

```
If the stain of the organism is grampos
```

```
and the morphology is coccus
and the growth conformation is chains
then there is suggestive evidence (0.7) that
the organism is streptococcus
```

Or, in the case of the simple nursing example:

```
If the patient is unconscious
and no pulse may be detected
then cardiopulmonary resuscitation is
required immediately
```

The application of rules to facts, by means of the software of the
expert system, generates new facts, such as:

```
There is suggestive evidence (0.7) that
Sample 7 is streptococcus
```

or

```
The patient in bed 7 requires immediate
cardiopulmonary resuscitation
```

The view of knowledge encouraged by expert systems is that of
knowledge rendered as facts (with all the implications of
categorization) and mechanistic rules (albeit more subtle and
complex than those of my simple illustration). It is a view of
expertise that regards professional expertise as rule-governed
behaviour that, *par excellence*, is both explicable and reproduc-
ible as planned, rational behaviour in attainment of explicit
goals. Furthermore, it is a view of expertise as a distinct and
separate product, capable of divorce from the expert who
displays it, which may be (re)produced as software on a
(potentially) vast number of machines, just like any other
industrial artefact. In this respect, it is noteworthy that expert
systems technology involves the use of *knowledge engineers*. A
knowledge engineer 'interviews the experts, organizes the
knowledge, decides how it may be represented in the expert
system ...' (Waterman, 1986, p.9). It is a view of knowledge
and expertise that assumes and promulgates expertise as a
uniform, standard and consistent activity.

Such a view of knowledge and expertise is not without
persuasion and appeal, yet it is a view that is a transformation
of the existing nature of professional expertise as revealed by
empirically-based studies. For example, Suchman (1987) has
shown that the human expertise displayed in the operation of
a photocopier system is not reducible to the systematic achievement of goals by rational plans. Leith (1986) has shown

that the application of rule-based expert systems to the legal process is a fatally flawed enterprise: legal expertise and the legal process are not the same as a system of facts and rules. Brody (1986, 1987), Lopez (1986) and Suchman (1987) have reported on behaviour that is clearly of a highly expert nature, yet, equally clearly, is not the simple application of rules and facts. These empirically-based studies all emphasize the situated and negotiated nature of expertise. That is to say, they emphasize expertise as, fundamentally, something displayed by experts, rather than being a distinct and separate commodity, as part of, and constituting, a particular social context.

As with the two previous paradigms, I would emphasize that I am not seeking to show that expert systems are 'wrong' in some technological or moral sense. Clearly, expert systems exist and computer technology has much to offer in terms of the sophisticated and complex interaction between rules and facts. Rather, I would seek to stress that the interaction between rules and facts, however sophisticated and complex, is not the same thing as expertise. This is not some subtle point of philosophy or a quibble over words: it is an intensely *practical* point. Leith expresses this issue of practicality when discussing an expert system to formalize the British Nationality Act of 1981: '... I can only reiterate the advice to potential immigrants or those concerned with their nationality to discuss the problem with an expert; not with a legal rule- or logic-based expert system. The advice they would get could not possibly be worse' (Leith, 1986, p.551). To ignore this advice is to accept that expert systems technology has transformed the nature of knowledge and expertise.

Postscript

In my discussion above, I have concentrated on three paradigms to illustrate the issues that arise with the representation and processing of knowledge through computer technology. There are, of course, more issues and more subtle complexities than those addressed in my treatment. A seminal text on this wider landscape is that of Weizenbaum (1984), whilst there are numerous papers examining specific issues. In particular, those of sociologists, psychologists and philosophers (as well as those of computer technologists) frequently offer revealing insights (see, for example, Hofstadter and Dennett, 1982; Woolgar, 1985; Winograd and Flores, 1986; Bloomfield,

1989). However, the same common theme runs through this work: that computer technology brings its own epistemological baggage and that any self-respecting user of such technology at least needs to be aware of the contents of that baggage.

References

Bloomfield, B.P. (1989) On speaking about computing. *Sociology*, 23 (3), 409–426

Boulanger, A.G. (1983) The expert system PLANT/cd: a case study in applying the general purpose inference system ADVISE to predicting black cutworm damage in corn. MSc Thesis, Department of Computer Science, University of Illinois

Brody H. (1986) *Maps and Dreams*, Faber and Faber, London

Brody, H. (1987) *Living Arctic*, Faber and Faber, London

Date, C.J. (1990) *An Introduction to Database Systems*, vol. 1, 5th edn, Addison-Wesley, Reading MA

Hofstadter, D. R. and Dennett, D. C. (1982) *The Mind's I*, Penguin, London

Jones, J. A. (1988) Clinical reasoning in nursing. *Journal of Advanced Nursing*, 13, 185–192

Kent, W. (1979) Limitations of record-oriented information models. *ACM Transactions on Database Systems*, 4, 1

Kuhn, T. S. (1970) *The Structure of Scientific Revolutions*, 2nd edn, University Press, Chicago

Leith, P. (1986) Fundamental errors in legal logic programming. *Computer Journal*, 29 (6), 545–552

Lopez, B. (1986) *Arctic Dreams*, Pan, London

Massie, S. (1988) Chips and nurses. *Senior Nurse*, 8 (9/10), 5–6

Mathiassen, L. and Andersen, P. B. (1983) Nurses and semiotics: the impact of EDP-based systems upon professional languages. *Sixth Scandinavian Research Seminar on Systemeering*

Robinson, H. M. (1989) *Database Analysis and Design*, 2nd edn, Chartwell-Bratt, Bromley

Robinson, K. S. M. (1986) The social construction of health visiting. PhD Thesis, Polytechnic of the South Bank, London

Shortliffe, E. H. (1976) *Computer-based Medical Consultations: MYCIN*, Elsevier, New York

Suchman, L. A. (1987) *Plans and Situated Actions*, University Press, Cambridge

von Grey, M. L. (1990) A look at the benefits of an integrated nursing system. *Information Technology in Nursing*, 2 (3), 40–41

Waterman, D. A. (1986) *A Guide to Expert Systems*, Addison-Wesley, Reading MA

Weizenbaum, J. (1984) *Computer Power and Human Reason*, Pelican, London

Windsor, P. (1986) *Introducing Körner*, BJHC Books, Weybridge

Winograd, T. and Flores, F. (1986) *Understanding Computers and Cognition: A New Foundation for Design*, Ablex, Norwood, New Jersey

Woolgar, S. (1985) Why not a sociology of machines? The case of sociology and artificial intelligence. *Sociology*, **19** (4), 557–572

Chapter 13

The politics of knowledge

Kate Robinson

What types of knowledge should nurses use? How much of the knowledge base of nursing should be scientific, or can be scientific? These are the kinds of question which have exercised the minds of the nursing leadership for at least two or three decades. The relationship between nursing and scientific knowledge has been particularly central to the discussion. This relationship can be manifested in at least two ways. First, nursing knowledge can itself be seen as scientific knowledge, at least in part; indeed a major thrust within the nursing educational system for the last twenty years has been the message that nursing is, or needs to become, a science. And scientific knowledge also makes a contribution to nursing knowledge in the form of knowledge derived from other disciplines which are part of the P2000 nursing curriculum (the curriculum approved for nursing courses at Diploma in Higher Education level and above). These 'external' disciplines include biology, sociology, psychology, chemistry, etc. The idea that nursing knowledge would 'mine' these external disciplines, and that teachers in those areas would have to be discipline experts rather than nurses with some knowledge of the discipline, was a central tenet of P2000 curriculum planning.

Over the decades the debate has moved in different directions. In the 1970s, for example, Hall, in Canada, was berating nurses for not being sufficiently scientific (Hall, 1970); similarly in England, MacFarlane was urging nurses to become more rational and scientific (MacFarlane, 1977). However, by the beginning of the 1990s we find increasing concern about emphasizing the 'art' in nursing to complement the 'science'.

For example, a series of seminars held by the Institute of Nursing, Oxford, in 1991 was entitled *Explorations in the Art and Science of Caring*, and many of the contributions were concerned about a philosophical rather than a scientific approach to nursing care. It is easy to let the extraordinariness of such a title go unremarked. Its very mundane effectiveness draws upon a rhetoric where discussion of a whole range of philosophical, intuitive and (for want of a better label) 'alternative' therapies becomes neither provocative nor bizarre.

So, questions about the nature and function of science are extremely important in nursing. However, in order to make sensible decisions about the incorporation of science into nursing or the mutation of nursing knowledge itself into science, we need to know the value of scientific knowledge; to explore whether the knowledge produced by scientific work is 'skewed' or 'flawed' in some way. If that were found to be so, then obviously the conclusions which are drawn from it in relation to nursing care may be unsafe in both a physical and conceptual sense. Discussions about these issues can be found in the nursing literature, but they have mainly focused on an exploration of the epistemological issues (see, for example, Orr, 1979). But there is also a more fundamental dimension or critique which we need to address in order to understand how compatible science is with the kind of values and goals which are espoused by nursing. We need to be able to answer the question: 'Are science and nursing compatible bedfellows?'

This might seem to be a strange question to those of you raised on the idea that science is a neutral, value-free process – an anodyne technique for the production of truths. Such is the view of science which is often presented to nursing students. That is to say, it is one which offers a bland, uncritical view of scientific work as adhering to a number of criteria. These criteria include the ideas, for example, that science is neutral or value free; that scientific knowledge is inherently superior to other forms of knowledge; that there is a single and objective reality, which may be discovered by the correct application of *the* scientific method. This account of science is derived largely from a Whig history of the natural sciences: that is, one which emphasizes the importance of the actions of 'great' individuals and the inevitability of progress (see Chapter 2). It is well expressed in a lecture given by George Steiner (Steiner, 1989), in which he attributes the growth of science to the masculine desire to pursue abstract truth; what he calls 'speculative lust'. It is, he suggests, a peculiarly male characteristic and an individualistic pursuit which has its roots in Ancient Greek culture. He cites (Steiner, 1989, p.184) the example of Archimedes:

> When Syracuse was captured in 212 BC, invading soldiers broke into Archimedes' garden. His mechanical devices had kept the assailants at bay. Now they were out for blood. Bent over a problem in the geometry of conic sections, Archimedes did not hear his killers coming. He perished, as it were, in a fit of abstraction.

Here, then, is the picture of the individual, detached from society about him, devoted to abstract thought. It is a very powerful image of science, a kind of *Boys' Own* comic view of how scientists work, although if Archimedes were working today we would expect him to be in a white coat in a laboratory.

Such ideas of science are perpetuated within nursing (and elsewhere) through a number of sources. First, from the contributions to the curriculum made by lecturers in specialized subjects: biologists, chemists, psychologists, etc. These are likely to be normatively inclined; that is to say, they will present a picture of their subject which emphasizes the reasonableness and normalness of both its methods and findings. While some well-known controversies may be included in the curriculum, a complex discussion of the fundamental epistemological and political problems of the discipline is likely to be avoided. Many of the histories of such subjects are also Whig histories, woven round the names of the 'great men' of their subject, and paying little regard to the social and economic context in which work was done. Second, it is derived from the accounts of research – of scientific production work – to be found in nursing research textbooks. These usually emphasize that scientific work is a straightforward process or 'recipe' which can be pursued in an unproblematic way by suitable motivated individuals (see, for example, Cormack, 1984; Clark and Hockey, 1989; Couchman and Dawson, 1990). Even an excellent textbook on research such as *Nursing Research: The Application of Qualitative Approaches* (Field and Morse, 1985) deals only with the complexities of what we may call 'micro-issues'; it neglects the macro-issues of the relationship between research and society. This is a particularly surprising omission as proponents of qualitative research have suffered greatly from the attacks of normative scientists.

How far is this an accurate picture of the reality of science and scientific work? The view of science as an individualistic activity carried out somehow 'outside' of society, and as scientists divorced from the realities of living within a particular time and space, has been increasingly subject to critical re-evaluation. Steiner (1989) suggests that the critique of science is as old as science itself and comes from four sources:

- Mystical
- Religious–dogmatic
- Romantic–existentialist
- Relativist or dialectical.

However, he acknowledges a more recent fifth and more fundamental critique (Steiner, 1989, p.190):

> But now, and for the first time in man's history, there is a new and total challenge to the ideal of the hunt after pure, abstract truth. For the first time, one can conceive of a fundamental incongruence, of a fundamental coming out of phase, between the pursuit of truth and equally demanding ideals of social justice or, even more centrally, between truth and survival.

At last we find science linked to its products, to its effects on society. Indeed, if we look back at the reference to Archimedes earlier in this chapter it is clear that such a link is obvious, although Steiner uses the account for a very different purpose. But if you read the quotation again, the most striking thing for me is the fact that Archimedes' 'abstract' thinking had clearly led directly to improvements in weaponry!

Such a link between science and its products has been widely acknowledged in recent years; indeed it would be hard to ignore. However, it is often argued that there is nothing wrong with science as such, rather that it is misused. This position, often known in shorthand as the 'use and abuse' argument, is perhaps best articulated by Medawar (1989, p.148), a brilliant scientist and writer on science:

> There is, of course, a sense in which science and technology can be arraigned for devising new instruments of warfare, but another and more important sense in which it is the height of folly to blame the weapon for the crime. I would rather put it this way: in the management of our affairs we have too often been bad workmen, and like all bad workmen we blame our tools.

However, many of the current critiques of science go a great deal further than that. They do not allow the distinction between science and technology to absolve scientists of the responsibility for the consequences of science. Indeed, they would argue that science is intimately connected with the economic, political and military institutions of society and constantly interacting with them. More specifically, they argue that the political and social consequences of science are fundamental to the *genesis* of scientific knowledge as well as to the effects and consequences of that knowledge. Let us look more closely at such critiques.

The radical critique of science

Rose (1987) argues that the re-evaluation of science is linked to the critical thinking of the 1960s and 1970s:

> The challenge to the claimed neutrality of science reached new levels in the late sixties in the context of the anti-war movement and the rise of student protest. Science in the hands of the US government in Indochina, far from being progressive, appeared as an agent of the most repressive imperialism; in the ripples of the Cultural Revolution, authority was questioned, expertise denied, the elitism and hierarchy which the laboratory practice of science typifies were under attack. As the seventies wore on, the very status of scientific knowledge as the only sure way of obtaining approximations to true descriptions of the material world, began to be denied both within the radical science movement and by the relativist sociologists and philosophers.

There is thus a major challenge to the idea of a 'neutral' science, uninfluenced by class, race, nationality or politics; it was no longer seen as the abstract accumulation of knowledge – of facts, theories and techniques – which could be 'used' or 'abused' by society. When the 1960's activists looked at science, they found that, far from being 'outside' of society, the scientific world mirrored society. Those in charge of this 'neutral' science were overwhelmingly white, male and occupying privileged positions in advanced industrial society. The organization of scientific work was hierarchical and discriminatory. Scientific work was organized to produce profits or generate weapons of mass destruction.

Who are the critics? According to Rose (1987), they are people from the peace movement, feminists, ecologists and animal liberationists. Clearly such groups are offering different types of critique but the various foci of criticism can be brought together into a fairly coherent account of the problems, or as Rose suggests, the limits of science. Of course, Rose is himself a scientist (Professor of Biology at the Open University) so it is also clear that these debates and critiques are not merely external to science, but part of an internal debate. A central argument concerns the interrelatedness between science and political economy, specifically the link with Western capitalism and, by implication, imperialism. A further, related issue is the connection between scientific knowledge and prevailing ideologies of ruling elites. An example of this is scientific ideas about women, which have consistently mirrored and justified an ideology of male supremacy.

Political economy

Despite the image of the individual scientist toiling long hours to pursue a personal interest in abstract knowledge, the real image of modern science is the substantial industrial organization, tied to the state and to the needs of industry, as in, for example, a modern drug company. It is perhaps unsurprising that science is closely linked to the military–industrial needs of society. Much of the boost to modern science came during World War II when scientific work was linked to the mobilization of society in the process of total war. The obvious examples from that era are, of course, the development of the atomic bomb and of missile technology, but there are others: for example, the development of penicillin was closely linked to the war effort. As Ravetz (1979) comments: 'Science gets the credit for penicillin; society takes the blame for the Bomb.' But both developments were generated by teams of scientists working within the military–industrial framework of societies at war. The consequence of the pattern of scientific funding laid in the war has been an enormous concentration on research into nuclear fission and fusion and radioastronomy (largely derived from techniques of radar). The major new initiative has been the Alvey programme, which was funded in the 1980s to promote research into computing. The programme was intended to ensure the survival of the UK computer industry into the next century despite enormous competition from Japanese industrial research and development initiatives.

Scientific work today is usually extremely expensive and those who fund it, that is, the state and powerful multinational corporations, expect it to serve their interests. The alliance between modern science and the state is not a new one and was certainly present by the end of the last century, if not earlier. This has created an industrialized science which is closely bound up with technology: that is, the practical application of scientific work. The 'idealized' description of science which separates it from its application through technology is probably related more closely to a model of science found in the universities than in industry. Richards (1983), for example, in the context of scientists working in the aircraft industry and nuclear power, writes:

> These individuals are, in the broadest and most realistic sense, all working in applied science; only an arbitrary distinction could separate them into scientists on the one hand and technologists on the other.

What is clear about such individuals is that they are subject to motives and pressures which are very different from those of the relatively protected world of the universities. Not only are the traditional distinctions between science and technology, basic and applied science, broken down, but even that between established and specific academic disciplines may be unclear in the pervading atmosphere of inter-disciplinary collaboration for the good of the firm. How does the difference in work environment affect attitudes to work? Does the applied scientist feel a commitment to norms that are different from those of the idealized ethos of science, or of a particular research network?

Of course, things are not as they were in the university sector either. Laboratories find themselves designated as 'cost centres', forced to prostitute themselves with whatever sponsors they can find in order to survive.

Ideology

Rose (1987) argues that science is ideologically bounded in three ways. First, only certain questions can be asked within science. Second, not all scientific 'facts' are considered to be of equal value. Third, scientists have adopted reductionism as both a central method and as a philosophy, and this limits their perspective: for example, it cannot cope with ecology. As illustration, he offers a useful example of two answers to the question 'Why did the frog's leg twitch?' The first answer, *'because of the effect of motor impulses on the muscle'*, clearly belongs to the reductionist tradition, and, while useful, offers a limited account of 'because'. The second possible answer, *'because the frog was jumping to escape a predator'*, may also be useful, but requires a more holistic interpretation of the word 'because'.

The difficulty we have in appreciating the ideological nature of a scientist's answer, which obviously provides for more than one 'correct' answer to a scientific question, is illustrated by the text from the Windscale inquiry. Collins (1985) suggests that lawyers find it difficult to appreciate that scientists may reach different conclusions based on fundamental differences of ideological perspective. For example, Justice Parker saw the disagreements between scientists about the evidence as accusations of dishonesty rather than different interpretations of evidence governed by different values. He defended (cited in Collins, 1985, p.161) the government scientists:

> I have no doubt as to the integrity of those concerned in all of [the controlling authorities] and I regard the attacks made upon them as without foundation.

The social sciences

Although I have so far largely illustrated the text with examples from the natural sciences, the social sciences must share the general critique, even if they differ in epistemological viewpoint. The link between science and the ruling élites of the state and industry is not confined to the natural sciences. Dorothy Smith (1988) argues that the function of sociology has been to map out those areas of life which are of interest to the ruling élites. Specifically, she argues that the way in which sociology is organized is dictated by the way in which the ruling élite defines its own relationships. For example, as they define women's work as unimportant, so sociologists have ignored it (with a few notable exceptions: see, for example, Gavron, 1966; Oakley, 1976; Delamont, 1980). Similarly, the organizations which are important to the ruling élite, such as the educational system, have formed the main topics of interest to sociologists, who have offered an increased under-standing of how these work. Such an argument can explain why nursing research is relatively underfunded. Smith argues further that we need to acknowledge that even the ways in which sociologists think is related to, or dictated by, the rulers or successful groups within our society.

The way in which sociology is organized therefore, according to Smith's critique, offers no place to the subject, no voice to those who are not part of or who are rendered impotent by the ruling élite. If we consider which categories of people are excluded from ruling in our society, it is obvious that sociology, and by implication science in general, excludes the categories of women, the lower classes, and in some situations, black people from participation in the production of scientific or valid knowledge.

The feminist critique

The feminist critique, in particular, links the two issues of political economy and ideology. It has been argued by many feminists that science is a male preserve and that scientific findings further male interests in producing findings which favour male dominance (in psychology, for example). Further, they argue that women are largely excluded from the interesting jobs in science and that where they do make important contributions these are disregarded. A prime example of this is the work of Rosalind Franklin which contributed enormously to the discovery of the structure of DNA but which has been largely ignored in the writing of the history and the receipt of the plaudits.

Science, they argue, has been concerned with understanding nature in order to manipulate and control it, and with the industrial processes of production, rather than with the natural processes of reproduction. Where scientists have turned their attention to human life and reproduction, it is with an industrial model in mind and the intent is to manipulate and change. The Brighton Women and Science Group, for example, have looked critically at areas of scientific work, such as contraception, mental health, childbirth, psychological testing, etc., to see how science relates to women (see Brighton Women and Science Group, 1980; Sayers, 1982).

The remedy?

There are at least two different positions within the feminist critique: either that science is so corrupt that it must be abandoned entirely as an endeavour, or that science can be reformed to take into account the criticisms. The degree to which the latter may be possible depends on the analysis of the cause of the problem.

Steiner (1989, p.195), for example, argues that science has grown big and complex merely because of 'pragmatic and technical reasons': that is, 'demanded' by the questions, which are derived in his scheme from the 'sceptical lust' of individuals:

> 'Big science' is no accidental outcome of megalomania. It is inherent in the internal development of physics, of chemistry, of molecular biology, of astronomy and astrophysics. Collaborative ... research and large scale instrumentation have sprung inevitably out of the nature of the problems to be solved.

Clearly such an explanation will not do. It neglects entirely the industrialization of science and the major sources of funding in the state, in particular the military, and private corporations. Questions do not 'spring out of' problems. People construct questions and problems in particular kinds of ways in response to what they, or their employers, see as important.

And nursing?

It seems to me that there is a danger that nursing will move from one extreme position to another, each equally illogical. In the 1960s and 1970s influential sectors of the occupation were committed to the 'scientization' of nursing. In the 1980s and 1990s that position is shifting, but not to a more complex consideration of how nursing might relate to scientific work. Instead, there is an 'anti-science' movement which is in danger of throwing out the baby with the bathwater. If you are tempted to live without science I would suggest that you attempt to care for your patients for one day without the benefit of a light bulb! We must acknowledge that science is intricately linked with the society in which it exists; but that must also be true, of course, of every other type of knowledge. To suppose that nursing knowledge of any sort can ever be 'value free' or can encompass values too far removed from those of the ruling élite of society is the ultimate arrogance.

What is important is that we are aware of the links between our knowledge and the society in which we live.

References and further reading

Bliss, M. (1982) *The Discovery of Insulin*, Faber and Faber, London

Brighton Women and Science Group (1980) *Alice Through the Microscope*, Virago, London

Clark, J.M. and Hockey, L. (1989) *Further Research for Nursing*, Scutari, London

Collins, H.M. (1985) *Changing Order: replication and induction in scientific practice*, Sage

Cormack, D.F.S. (ed.) (1984) *The Research Process in Nursing*, Blackwell, Oxford

Couchman, W. and Dawson, J. (1990) *Nursing and Health Care Research*, Scutari, London

Delamont, S. (1980) *The Sociology of Women*, Allen and Unwin, London

Field, P.A. and Morse, J.M. (1985) *Nursing Research: The Application of Qualitative Approaches*, Chapman and Hall, London

Gavron, H. (1966) *The Captive Wife*, Penguin, Harmondsworth

Goldberg, J. (1988) *Anatomy of a Scientific Discovery*, Bantam, London

Hall, O. (1970) Social change, specialization, and science: where does nursing stand? In *Nursing Education in a Changing Society* (ed. M.Q. Innis), University Press, Toronto

MacFarlane, J.K. (1977) Developing a theory of nursing: the relation of theory to practice. *Journal of Advanced Nursing*, 2(3), 261–270

Medawar, P. (1989) On 'The effecting of all things possible', from Pluto's Republic, 1982, In *From Creation to Chaos* (ed. B. Dixon), Blackwell, Oxford

Nowatny, H. and Rose, H. (eds) (1979) *Counter-Movements in the Sciences*, D. Reidel, London

Oakley, A. (1976) *Housewife*, Penguin, Harmondsworth

Orr, J.A. (1979) Nursing and the process of scientific enquiry. *Journal of Advanced Nursing*, 4, 603–610

Ravetz, J. (1979) Anti-establishment science in some British journals. In *Counter-Movements in the Sciences* (eds H. Nowatny and H. Rose), D. Reidel, London

Richards, S. (1983) *Philosophy and Sociology of Science*, Blackwell, Oxford

Robinson, K. (1985) Knowledge and its relationship to health visiting. In *Health Visiting* (eds K. Lukor and J. Orr), Blackwell, Oxford

Rose, H. (1987a) Making science feminist. In *The Changing Experience of Women* (eds E. Whitelegge *et al.*), Martin Robertson, Oxford

Rose, S. (1987b) *Molecules and Minds*, Open University Press, Milton Keynes

Sayers, J. (1982) *Biological Politics*, Tavistock, London

Smith, D. (1988) *The Everyday World as Problematic: A Feminist Sociology*, Open University Press, Milton Keynes
Steiner, G. (1989) Has truth a future? Bronowski Memorial Lecture 1978. In *From Creation to Chaos* (ed. B. Dixon) Blackwell, Oxford, pp. 189–197

Chapter 14

Knowing nursing: emerging paradigms in nursing

Alan Pearson

As other chapters in this book have shown, the construction of knowledge stems from the paradigm which underpins its construction. Following Kuhn (1970), a paradigm is the 'entire constellation of beliefs, values, techniques', and so on shared by the community. This chapter builds on Part One of this book, exploring the nature of knowing nursing, and emerging paradigms which appear to be appropriate for theorizing or generating new knowledge in nursing.

On knowing nursing

Nursing, as a collective, frequently misses the point of its very existence: the provision of a nursing service to those who need, seek, or are directed to, nursing. Jacox (1974) purports that practice, or service delivery, is the alpha and omega of nursing, and all else which surrounds or cloaks practice is meaningless in comparison to it. Nursing is, quite simply, a practice, but its practice is far from simple. In fact, so complex is our practice, that, to date, we know very little as an occupation about its subtleties. Yet our expert practitioners and expert patients know a great deal, but we have paid too little attention to unlocking the knowledge they hold in their heads. As Schön (1983) says, expert nurses know far more than they can ever tell.

What do we really mean by 'knowing nursing'? Nurses all share the common heritage of living as, and being, a nurse.

This in itself gives us insights and biases, and a unique sort of knowing about the world of health care and the clients and health workers which provide its population. All nurses *know* nursing, though *what* they know may be different, and *how* they know and perceive their knowing is different. This is dependent on many things, not least the unique experiences of the nurse and the nurse's own desire and ability to reflect upon experience. *Knowing*, or *to know*, is defined in the Macquarie Dictionary (1988) as: 'to perceive or understand as fact or truth; or apprehend with clearness and certainty.' Logical and commonsensical though this definition is, it tells us little about nursing knowledge, or how it is acquired. Carper (1978), in her attempt to explicate patterns of knowing in nursing, is perhaps a little more helpful. She suggests that there are four such patterns: ethical, empirical, aesthetic and personal (see Chapter 1).

Knowing nursing, then, perhaps incorporates all four of these forms of knowledge, and more. Most of us probably realize that we 'know' in these four forms, yet the knowledge we possess as persons is not necessarily knowledge which is available and accessible to the occupation as a whole. In other words, nurses know on an *individual* level, yet nursing does not, as yet, know on a *collective* level. We have failed to make our knowledge as individuals open to others. In doing this, we have also put up barriers to finding out more. Only when we understand what we know, and the limitations of our knowledge, will we be able to generate more knowledge through testing and refining. Personal and practical knowledge (the latter, of course, being a part of Carper's conception of personal knowledge, though it is somewhat underemphasized by her) are perhaps the strongest patterns of knowing in contemporary nursing. Yet we have undersold the importance and sophistication of these two ways of knowing, as well as neglecting the development of other patterns.

Furthermore, we have not always wanted to know nursing in its fullest sense, nor encouraged those who do want to know. Historically, nursing has often devalued those who really want to *know nursing*, and has overvalued those who wish to be proficient in *carrying out the tasks of nursing*, regarding nursing knowledge as static. Nursing's development over the past fifty years has also been overly influenced by other disciplines, overvaluing those which support nursing, such as the physical sciences, sociology and psychology. While the tasks of nursing, and the disciplines which are drawn on to support it are important areas of knowledge to nurses, they do not constitute *nursing knowledge*. An overconcentration on them hinders our ability to really understand the practice discipline of nursing itself.

Attempts to grapple with nursing and to understand it more fully have been made in relatively recent times; nurses themselves have engaged in explicit theorizing about their own discipline. Theorizing, or thinking about nursing itself, is nothing more than attempting to articulate what we know of nursing, or to map out nursing knowledge.

The theoretical development of nursing: articulating nursing knowledge

The theoretical development of nursing has, it is often claimed, been limited and unsophisticated until recent times. Many commentators suggest that real successes in developing theoretical understandings of our discipline have only occurred within the past thirty years. This chapter is, to some extent, an attempt to clarify and challenge these widely held assumptions.

Rogers (1983) addresses the future of nursing, and urges us: 'to glimpse a becoming, to see with that "third eye" ... to speculate upon a dream and to watch that dream unfold ... to create a new reality.' My field of vision is, I fear, somewhat limited and I do not claim to be able to see through the 'third eye' described by Rogers; I cannot see beyond the horizon, but I can see a range of different views. Nor do I claim to be an authority on nursing theory, as I, like many nurses, am still struggling to understand various horizons, and to find a position which is comfortable. This chapter is a 'thinking out aloud' endeavour of someone who is still a student of the discipline.

I am quintessentially a nurse and carry with me the inheritance of nursing past and all that entails: an understanding of nursing that stems from a commitment to service, a valuing of doing, a burdening of concrete thinking and pragmatism which sometimes overwhelms my desire to be scholarly, and a tendency to devalue all that is classically theoretical. I know this: and struggle with my inheritance daily in my work. But I also recognize the importance of myself being a nurse, and try to use this part of me in my own search to understand nursing. Martha Rogers (1983) asserts that:

'Those who seek to perpetuate the past, no matter how well-meaning they may be are destined to fall by the wayside. They will not cross the horizon.' My reply is that those who denigrate the past and deny nursing's inheritance may well cross the one horizon they see in front of them but, in so doing, may never see the multiplicity of horizons available to them by simply looking at the real world of nursing as they turn slowly through 360° and reflect on the views.

'Theorizing nursing' is perhaps a rather pompous way of saying 'thinking about nursing', and the mystery of nursing to be discovered is about who we are. Our lives as nurses, and my living as a nurse, are perhaps the process through which this discovery occurs. This chapter serves as a means by which I can share some of my tentative thinking about nursing.

Theory and theorizing in nursing

Currently, nursing is energetically interested in theory of, for or in nursing. So what does the world conventionally mean by the word theory?

Theory is a formulation of ideas; a conceptualization of the real with the purpose of comprehending it fully. Clearly, theory arises through human thinking and this process of thinking about phenomena (and possibly experimentation on, or manipulation of, the world to confirm such thinking) is what is meant by theorizing. Indeed, Kaplan (1964) says that theory formation or theorizing is an important and distinctive attribute of all human beings. It is a human characteristic and ability, and a process which is not removed from experience. Both theorizing and experience are inextricably linked to each other. Dickoff, James and Wiedenbach (1986) assert that: 'theoretically speaking, anyone capable of speech is potentially capable of theorising.'

The human characteristic of theorizing has undoubtedly been a feature of nursing throughout the ages. Knowledge development and theorizing in nursing has passed through a series of influences since the advent of Nightingale. Initially, it was rooted in medical knowledge, and this prevailed until the late 1940s to early 1950s, when nurses entered courses in education in large numbers, leading to a bias towards educational knowledge and processes in theorizing nursing. Soon after this, nurses also began to study other disciplines, and their theory began to influence theorizing in nursing. In the mid-1960s, a concentration on conceptual systems developed and attempts to articulate grand theories appeared. Only recently has nursing begun to theorize from a practice–theory position, using epistemological positions rather than grand theory positions.

Conflicting views of theory and theorizing in nursing

Having briefly suggested how nursing's theorizing has developed, it is appropriate now to turn to current debates on theory and to relate this to nursing.

Tripp (1987) argues that theory does not have a single, simple meaning, and that there are different 'kinds' of theory: for example, grand theory, critical theory personal theory, local theory, normative theory, practical theory and espoused theory. He suggests that these different kinds of theory can be loosely grouped into epistemological theories, grand theories, local theories and metatheories.

Epistemological theories transcend specific disciplinary boundaries and seek to perceive and investigate the world. Grand theories are concerned with understanding particular features of the world and are therefore specific to a particular discipline. Local theories relate to a particular context and are therefore quite specific to a particular place and time. Metatheories are concerned with the nature, generation and use of theory itself.

The literature suggests that such a broad view of what theory and theorizing is, is only just emerging in nursing. There seems to have been a preoccupation with grand theory, and scant attention paid to local theory. Furthermore, the only respectable sort of theorizing has been seen as that which fits the natural and physical sciences, and therefore focuses on distance from action and the world of practice. Theorizing associated with the development of theoretical knowledge has become regarded as that which generates real theory, whereas theorizing associated with action has come to be seen as 'non-theory', or even as the opposite of theory.

Walker (1971), for example, suggests that there are three categories of theorizing: applied/basic, theoretical and practical. She argues, however, that practical theorizing is best categorized as praxiology, and thus cannot be truly related to theory, since theory is 'typically employed in the context of systematic description and explanation'. She argues that practice theory is grounded in principles of action, and action-oriented endeavours are not conventionally regarded as theory. This assertion follows the conception that what is *not* the doing is *theory.*

Following this line of argument, praxiology and the principles of practice, says Walker, lead to rules for carrying out nursing as a process, but theory provides knowledge about the process. Although it is often claimed that observation of clinical practice is a wellspring for theory development, Walker disputes this, arguing that such a claim is epistemologically inadequate as it confuses nursology (theoretical knowledge) with practical knowledge.

Rogers (1983) asserts that:

> A firm belief in nursing as an organized body of abstract knowledge arrived at by scientific research and logical analysis is an essential pre-requisite to nurses' ability to serve people knowledgeably.... The practice of nursing derives from nursing's body of scientific knowledge specific to nursing.

She argues that current efforts to confront *practice* theorizing and *theoretical* theorizing to develop theory through such approaches as unification and joint appointments are merely a reversion to apprenticeship training and an attempt to maintain the status quo, and confuse practice with theory. Many nurse scholars concur with this and seem to agree with the sentiment 'When ideals sink to the level of practice, stagnation is the result'.

Others disagree with this notion of separating theory and practice, arguing that nursing, as a practice discipline, is logically intensely interested in practice. The need for the theorizing of nursing by both practitioners and scholars of nursing is central to understanding nursing, and a preoccupation with traditionally defined notions of theory is invalid in such a field. Street (1988) asks, for example:

> Given that the aim of the theorist was to explain, predict and organize knowledge about nursing practice, how did the practice discipline of nursing develop along a theoretical road which has created a dichotomy between nursing theory and the reality of clinical practice?

She argues that the adoption of a positivist paradigm has led to this dichotomy. Smyth (unpublished observations, 1986) purports that this dichotomy is unnecessary, arguing that:

This separation is given a form of pseudo-legitimacy in scholarly and academic circles, as well as in the language with which we speak about facets of everyday life. There is a widespread view that while theory is one thing, practice is quite different. I want to suggest that theory and practice should not be thought of as being opposed to one another. In a very real sense there is an interpenetration of the two; that is to say, elements each exist in the other. By continuing to insist on:

- the translation of theory into practice
- closing the gap between theory and practice
- integrating theory and practice

we are still fundamentally wedded to the idea that theory and practice are separate.

This contrasts starkly with Walker's (1971) views. She suggests that in order to answer the question 'What is nursing?' three sub-questions need to be posed:

- What is occurring in nursing?
- What is effective nursing?
- What is worthwhile nursing?

What occurs in nursing is, she suggests, best addressed in the scientific mode, and what is worthwhile in nursing, in the philosophic. The question of what is effective nursing lies, she argues, in the area of praxiology, and thus is not theoretical. To confuse praxiology and practical knowledge with nursology or theoretical knowledge will lead to theory being made to serve the more narrow and immediate purposes of practice. Wooldridge (1971) disagrees vehemently with Walker's position. He argues that what is occurring and what is worthwhile cannot be properly regarded as nursing theory at all, nor can theorizing about them be nursing theorizing as such. Such 'theories about nursing' are nursing theories only in the sense that nurses are the subject matter to be investigated. He argues that it is practice theories, and thus practical theorizing, that are the special province of nursing. It is perhaps easier to forge an allegiance with one of these alternative positions, and to vehemently defend it. To reject the other leads to a position of relative certainty.

A more challenging option is to acknowledge the existence of both, and to appreciate the merits and shortcomings of each. To do so in nursing is apparently difficult because of our heritage and the tendency to compartmentalize thinking from doing. This may be compounded by the pervasive valuing of the theory–practice dichotomy, and the relative paucity of discussion about practice. For this reason, I want to turn to the less explored area of practice action: nursing's purpose for being.

Theorizing in action: the emerging paradigm to uncover nursing knowledge

Practice theory and praxiology relates to action, practical knowledge and theorizing. It is derived from the term praxis, variously defined as: 'a customary mode of behaviour: doing' (Longman English Dictionary); 'the general theory of efficient action' (Walker, 1971); and 'the action and reflection of people upon their world in order to transform it' (Friere, 1972).

Few would argue with the statement that practice is the *raison d'être* of nursing and that practice is grounded in action. Carr and Kemmis (1987) say that:

> A Practice . . . is not some kind of thoughtless behaviour which exists separately from theory and to which theory can be applied. Furthermore, all practices, like all observations, have theory embedded in them and this is just as true for the practice of theoretical pursuits as it is for those of practical pursuits. . . .

Nurses could no more nurse without reflecting upon (and, hence, theorizing about) what they are doing than theorists could produce theories without engaging in the sort of practices distinctive of their activity.

Commenting on their field of education, Carr and Kemmis argue that educational theory should reject positivist notions of rationality, objectivity and truth, accept the need to apply the interpretive categories of teachers, and provide ways of identifying distorted interpretations from those that are not. It must also provide some view of how any distorted self-understanding is to be overcome, be concerned to identify and expose obstacles presented by the prevailing social order which frustrate the pursuit of rational goals, and offer theoretical accounts which make teachers aware of how they may be eliminated or overcome, recognizing that theory is practical. Theorizing is not limited to those to whom we usually ascribe the term 'theorist'. As Sprinthall (1980) says, practice is not a 'second class activity for those too stupid to think at a theoretical level.' Practitioners theorize, and thus develop theories.

Ellis (1969) characterizes practitioners as theorists who select and restructure theories and test them in practice. She says that:

> ... we theorize without knowing we do it ... We are not sufficiently conscious of the extent to which we use theory in practice, nor of the extent to which we adapt theory in practice.

For example, nurses can often sense deterioration in a person before explicit signs appear, and often this conflicts with the perception of doctors. In some way, the nurse has developed an ability to identify certain tacit signs, and thus has attained a different theoretical stance from the doctor's. This theory in action is not explicit, and nurses are often not conscious of their own theorizing and resulting theoretical framework. This may be partly due to the clinician's interest in the goal of providing nursing, rather than in its analysis; the focus is on action itself, and not on its analysis

Ellis posits that a major reason for our failure to make such theory explicit is that:

> ... we may overlook the familiar, or perhaps devalue it. There is some danger of neglecting, or even rejecting some of the traditional, familiar components in nursing as we grow in our emphasis on science and research ... It is the professional practitioner who is able to criticize the theory in use and determine its value for directing actions to achieve desired outcomes. In this she is not only a user of theory, but she may be a modifier as well. She is also a chooser of theory.

Tripp (1987) argues for professional practitioners working towards their 'own individually constructed and possibly idiosyncratic theoretical framework, rather than picking up a universal theoretical framework ready-made by others'.

To start with theory is alienating, for it leads to 'it's OK in theory, but it won't work in practice' statements. However, starting in practice is equally problematic. People will only work on their own practice if they perceive a need to do so. But there must be implicit theories in practitioners' heads, and if they are empowered through reflection, and articulate their practice, they will be able to explicate their theories. Practitioners solve many problems every day because professional practice is a continuous process of professional judgement. Benner (1985) demonstrates the validity of this clearly in her explication of the knowledge embedded in expert practice. She says that:

> Expertise develops when the clinician tests and refines proposi-
> tions, hypotheses, and principle-based expectations in actual
> practice situations. Experience, as it is used here, results when
> preconceived notions and expectations are challenged, refined,
> or disconfirmed by the actual situation.

Is this not, then, theorizing?

> As a nurse gains experience, clinical knowledge that is a hybrid
> between naïve practical knowledge and unrefined theoretical
> knowledge develops.

Is this not, again, theorizing? This view of practice as a world of action, where practitioners engage in both practical and theoretical endeavour, begins, I believe, to open up a scene full of exciting possibilities.

Action

As our research and theorizing has become more sophisticated (at least in scientific terms), it may have held our eyes too long on a single view of theory or knowledge which is perceived to be valid. It has also become increasingly less useful for guiding our understanding of nursing practice. It is true to say, I believe, that much of our 'scholarly' theorizing is only dis-tantly related to the real world of practising nurses, especially when it utilizes the most rigorous methods of positivism, the mechanistic application of problem solving, or attempts to reduce and categorize the phenomena encountered in nursing.

These problems are best reflected in the prevailing concep-tion of theory as an accumulation of facts or concepts which can be drawn on by clinicians when they wish to apply them. This conception encourages our separation of theory from practice: our belief that theorizing relates only to the classical view of theory, and not thinking and reflecting. Published research, for example, is read more by the producers of research than by the practitioners whom we assume to be the rightful users. Consequently, the practitioners argue that the theorizing of nurse scholars lacks relevance and reflects a lack of interest in, or response to, the needs of practice. Further-more, the language used by scholars is not the language of nursing, which is rich in shared meaning to our practitioners and serves to encapsulate the knowledge embedded in expert practice (Benner, 1985).

This apparent issue of relevance, usefulness, or relatedness is perhaps more of an issue of epistemology. Scholarly nursing theorizing has espoused the positivistic model of science and its associated language. When this is applied to practice it often inadvertently undermines the values of practitioners, which are action-oriented and involve theorizing in action.

I would argue that a view which values theorizing which incorporates 'action', as well as action itself, would have the following qualities. It would:

- Look to the future, in that it seeks to transform.
- Value collaboration, in that it seeks to involve.
- Lead to development, in that it seeks to build and grow.
- Be concerned with generating theory grounded in action, rather than vice-versa.
- Be agnostic, in that it seeks to re-examine and reformulate, rather than to prescribe.
- Be situational, in that it seeks to recognize contexts and their full meanings.

A focus on action is legitimate, respectable and worthy of trust when theorizing nursing because, as a practice discipline, nursing is grounded in action.

Such an approach is rich in its opportunities for discovery. It is attractive to nursing and is philosophically familiar to nurses. Action-oriented theorizing and theory is perhaps the area we have least explored, despite our practice heritage. It offers, I believe, a vantage point from which to see multiple views which sit comfortably with the genesis and continuing ethos of nursing. It is the emerging paradigm of choice in nursing's search for knowledge. Gulino (1982) suggests that nursing's focus is on the person, and its concern lies in 'being'. Being is not, she argues, a problem to be mastered, but a mystery to be lived and we cannot merely study and explain a mystery. Mystery is not to be confused with the unknown or unknowable. It has a bearing on our lives; it arises out of our experience; and we have to deal with it by attitude and action: As Gulino (1982) says:

> Mystery assumes involvement and deep personal relationship, whereas problem solving demands a separation between myself and that which I am studying; abstraction; intellectualization; and generalization.

and:

> The nurse needs a heightened awareness of herself, an ability to live with the tentative, if she is not to be robbed of the reality of her own existence and that of her client.

She argues that investing in different ways of perceiving, of theorizing, and of knowing nursing and nursing-as-action will in time lead to the development of an understanding of nursing that encompasses the infinite possibilities of being human.

Although many of the questions in today's world are unanswerable, the ways in which nursing structures the questions, the provisional ways in which perspectives are formed, have significance for the evolution of the profession and thereby for the lives of our clients.

In theorizing nursing and in defining theory in nursing, perhaps we need to peruse the multiple horizons and to value them all: to perceive practical theory as legitimate theory; practice as theoretical; practitioners as theorists; and at the same time, to acknowledge those scholars whose expertise lies in developing theory from outside the practice world.

Conclusion

To conclude, knowing nursing and, thus, theorizing nursing, is many faceted and, though it has until recently had its vision fixed on the narrow horizon of traditional notions of knowledge, there are multiple horizons to view and discover. The whole constellation of this emerging paradigm can contribute to nursing's development, but we ought not deny the richness of practice by fixing our thoughts on any one view. We should be wary of theorists like Rogers (1983) who, in her vision of beyond the horizon in nursing, sees only one scene. It is a tripartite division of thinking/doing responsibilities, where:

> ... principles and theories generated by nursing's new paradigm engage scholars and scientists in nursing as they seek to push back the frontiers of knowledge. Nursing educators incorporate findings of nursing research into a rapidly growing body of substantial knowledge specific to nursing and transmit this knowledge to students seeking professional and technical careers in nursing. Practitioners of nursing translate this knowledge into novel and unexpected uses in their efforts to promote health and welfare.

If that is beyond the horizon, then I don't want to cross it. I want a world which gives me many views, and I want a world which acknowledges the action orientation of nursing, and the richness of theorizing alongside experience. I want to live in a world where there is a dialectical relationship between the theorizing and understandings of practitioners and scholars. I don't believe that the place across Rogers' horizon is a real world place; I don't believe that professional, action-people ever translate and use the theories generated by scholars and scientists, or that the knowledge transmitted by educators is the sole determinant of the future actions of the student. Some now claim that the future of nursing lies in recognizing the values and practices of the clinical practitioner. I concur wholeheartedly and will continue to keep turning around in my circle to see the views on the horizon which arise from the theorizing of scholars and practitioners. As Johann Wolfgang Von Goethe said in the eighteenth century:

All theory, dear friend, is grey, but the golden tree of life springs ever green.

References and further reading

Abdellah, F.G. and Levine, E. (1965) *Better Patient Care Through Nursing Research*, Macmillan, New York

Benner, P. (1985) *From Notice to Expert: Excellence and Power in Clinical Nursing Practice*, Addison–Wesley, Menlo Park CA

Bond, S. (1978) Dilemmas in clinical research. Paper presented at the *Northern Regional Health Authority Seminar on Developments in Nursing*, September.

Carper, B.A. (1978) Fundamental patterns of knowing in nursing, *Advances in Nursing Science*, **1(1)**, 13–23

Carr, W. and Kemmis, S. (1987) *Becoming Critical*, Deakin University Press, Victoria

Chinn, P. and Jacobs, M. (1987) *Theory and Nursing: A Systematic Approach*, Mosby, St Louis

Dickoff, J., James, P. and Wiedenbach E. (1986) Theory in a practice discipline. Part II: Practice oriented research. *Nursing Research*, **17(6)**, 545–554

Ellis, R. (1969) Practitioner as theorist. *American Journal of Nursing*, **69**, 1434–1438

Franklin, B. (1974) *Patient Anxiety on Admission to Hospital*, Royal College of Nursing, London

Friere, P. (1972) *Cultural Action for Freedom*, Penguin, London

Gulino, C.K. (1982) Entering the mysterious dimension of other: an existential approach to nursing care. *Nursing Outlook*, **30(6)**, 352–357

Jacox, A. (1974) Theory construction in nursing: an overview. *Nursing Research*, **23(1)**, 4–13

Kaplan, A. (1964) *The Conduct of Inquiry*, Chandler, New York

Kuhn, T.S. (1970) *The Structure of Scientific Revolutions*, 2nd edn, University of Chicago Press, Chicago

Longman English Dictionary (1976) Longman, London

McFarlane, J. (1980) *The Multi-Disciplinary Team*, King's Fund, London

Macquarie Dictionary (1988), 2nd edn, Macquarie Library, NSW, Australia

Meleis, A. (1985) *Theoretical Nursing: Development and Progress*, Lippincott, Philadelphia

Miller, A. (1985) The relation between nursing theory and nursing practice. *Journal of Advanced Nursing*, **10(5)**, 417–429

Pearson, A. (1985) The effects of introducing new norms in a nursing unit and an analysis of the process of change. PhD Thesis, Goldsmith's College, University of London

Pearson, A. (1987) Valuing and generating nursing knowledge. *Courage to Learn: Conference Proceedings*, Austin Hospital, Melbourne, pp.51–61.

Pearson, A. (1988) *Primary Nursing: Nursing in the Burford and Oxford Nursing Development Units*, Croom Helm, London

Rogers, M.E. (1983) Beyond the horizon. In *The Nursing Profession: A Time to Speak* (ed. N.L. Chaska), McGraw Hill, New York

Schon, D. A. (1983) *The Reflective Practitioner*, Basic Books, New York

Smyth, W.J. (1986) Peer clinical supervision as 'empowerment' versus 'delivery of a service'. Unpublished paper to AERA, San Francisco (April)

Sprinthall, N. (1980) Adults as learners. In *Exploring Issues in Teacher Education. Questions for Future Research* (eds G. Hall, S. Hurd and G. Brown), R and D Center for Teacher Education, University of Texas at Austin, pp.275–290

Street, A. (1988) Nursing practice: high, hard ground, messy swamps and the pathways in between. In *Reflective Processes in Nursing*, Faculty of Nursing Monograph Series, Deakin University Press, Victoria, pp.1–38

Treece, E.W. and Treece, J.W. (1980) *Elements of Research in Nursing*, Mosby, St Louis

Tripp, D. (1987) *Theorising Practice: The Teacher's Professional Journal*, Deakin University Press, Victoria

Walker, L.O. (1971) Toward a clearer understanding of the concept of nursing theory. *Nursing Research*, **20(5)**, 425–435

Wooldridge, P.J. (1971) Meta-theories of nursing: a commentary on Dr Walker's article. *Nursing Research*, **20(6)**, 445–495

Index